613.95

001916

ABC OF SEXUAL HEALTH

ABC OF SEXUAL HEALTH

edited by

JOHN TOMLINSON

Physician, Men's Health Clinic, Winchester
Formerly General Practitioner, Alton and Honorary Senior Lecturer in Primary Care,
University of Southampton

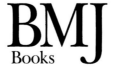

© BMJ Books 1999
BMJ Books is an imprint of the BMJ Publishing Group

First published in 1999
by BMJ Books, BMA House, Tavistock Square,
London WC1H 9JR
www.bmjbooks.com

British Library Cataloguing in Publication Data

A catalogue record for this book is available from the British Library

ISBN 0-7279-1373-5

Typeset by Apek Typesetters, Nailsea, Bristol
Printed and bound by Craft Print, Singapore

Contents

Contributors

Robin Bell, Staff Grade Physician in Genitourinary Medicine, St Mary's Hospital, London, UK

Josie Butcher, General Practitioner, Nantwich, Clinical Course Director of the MSc in Psychosexual Therapy, University of Central Lancashire, and Honorary Lecturer in Human Sexuality, Withington Hospital, Manchester, UK

Padmal de Silva, Consultant Clinical Psychologist, Senior Lecturer in Clinical Psychology, Institute of Psychiatry, Maudsley Hospital, London, UK

John Dean, General Practitioner who also runs a sexual dysfunction clinic, Plymouth, UK

Wallace Dinsmore, Consultant Physician, Royal Victoria Hospital, Belfast, UK

Asun de Marquiegui, Sex Therapist and Instructing Doctor in Family Planning, London, UK

Christine Evans, Consultant Urologist, Clwyd Hospital, Rhyl, UK

Clive Glass, Consultant Clinical Psychologist, North West Regional Spinal Injuries Unit, Southport District General Hospital, Southport, UK

Alain Gregoire, Consultant Psychiatrist, Old Manor Hospital, Salisbury, and Honorary Senior Lecturer, University of Southampton, UK

Christopher Headon, Psychotherapist, St George's Hospital, Whittington Hospital and the Albany Trust, and Instructor, Westminster Pastoral Foundation, London, UK

Margot Huish, Sex and Relationship Therapist, Barnet Healthcare NHS Trust, Barnet Hospital, London, UK

Roger Kirby, Consultant Urologist, St Bartholomew's Hospital, London, UK

Tony Parsons, Consultant Obstetrician and Gynaecologist, Rugby NHS Trust, and Senior Lecturer, University of Warwick, UK

Margaret Ramage, Tutor in Human Sexuality, St George's Hospital, London, Psychosexual Therapist, Wandsworth and Lambeth Health Authorities, UK

Jane Read, Author of "Counselling for infertility", and Sex and Relationship Therapist, London, UK

Bakulesh Soni, Consultant, North West Regional Spinal Injuries Unit, Southport District General Hospital, Southport, UK

John Tomlinson, Physician, Men's Health Clinic, Winchester. Formerly General Practitioner, Alton, and Honorary Senior Lecturer in Primary Care, University of Southampton, UK

Foreword

Individuals, the press and society, often find it difficult to handle and deal with sexual matters and sexual identity. The medical profession, as members of the public, will at times grapple with their own sexual orientation and problems, and have varying views and value systems around sexual matters and morality, and of course why not? They have a responsibility however to be well informed about sexual health so that they can educate and help patients at the same time as adopting a neutral and non-censorious position. It is bad manners and bad medicine to force one's own personal moral attitudes and beliefs about sexual matters on patients.

Sexual health is badly covered in the undergraduate curriculum, so doctors are not as knowledgeable and comfortable about this area of medicine to be of most help to their patients. In the light of this, the *ABC of Sexual Health* is to be warmly welcomed. The two current ABCs on *Sexually Transmitted Diseases* and *AIDS* have dealt primarily with the clinical aspects of these diseases. This new ABC is a much more detailed examination of sexual problems and variations. This only makes sense if done in an open and explicit fashion, and covers a wide variety of sexual habits and practices. Ultimately this approach will help us to understand a range of problems and behaviours so as to be able to deal with everyday issues presented by our patients. This book will put the profession in touch with the real world, real people with real problems, and fill a large gap in our knowledge.

Michael W. Adler
Professor of Sexually Transmitted Diseases
Department of Sexually Transmitted Diseases
Royal Free and University College Medical School
London

Preface

Although there are many sources of information on sex, presented with great openness and frankness, they are not necessarily accurate, and there has been a lack of authoritative information on sexuality and all its variations for medical and nursing students and for those practitioners who might come across sexual problems incidentally in their professional work. This collection of articles has attempted to fill a gap.

As a medical student, the only sex education that I had in my five years was a one hour lecture by the aged pioneer of contraception, Marie Stopes. The curiosity and thirst for information was huge, and the lecture hall was crammed to the doors. Later, when I was a course organiser for trainee general practitioners in the 1970s and 1980s, we asked the trainees what they would like to learn on the course.[1] Every term without exception, one of the most frequent requests was for help with psychosexual problems, as none of them had had any training in human sexuality. Unfortunately, with some notable exceptions, this still seems to be the case.

Equally, young people have little or no training in sexual health although they may know their human biology. Many parents find it difficult to talk to their children and research shows that there is enormous parental approval for schools to provide sex education, especially where it is done with their support. However, children themselves say that sex education is taught too late, often when puberty is well advanced and it focuses on biological aspects rather than on emotions and relationships, therefore not meeting their needs. One of the most consistent research findings is that earlier sex education does *not* increase sexual activity in young people. The Sex Education Forum[2] suggests that teaching should be started in primary school as part of the national curriculum and be ongoing through school life.

Our ambivalence and hyprocrisy towards sex results in a teenage pregnancy rate which is the worst in Europe and almost nine times that of Holland. In England and Wales alone in 1997, there were 8300 girls under 16 who became pregnant (including one ten year old and 158 aged 13 or under) and over half were aborted. From a medical and sociological stand point, this is unacceptable. Therefore, enabling the young to be more informed should eventually lead to a new generation of educated adults, including doctors, who can talk with ease about sexual matters, and who can feel comfortable about male and female emotions and relationships and I hope that the *ABC of Sexual Health* will make a contribution.

It was sad that there had to be a warning on the front of the Journal when these articles first appeared, about the sexually explicit material inside, a point emphasised in a letter to the Times.[3] Pictures of genital ailments are apparently acceptable, but an artist's picture showing the fun of sex needs a warning. Despite that warning, we did offend a very small number of readers. The illustrations could have been purely clinical photographs, but that would have been somewhat dull, and in any case, our sexual nature has been celebrated in explicit detail by all sorts of famous artists throughout history. We had choices from painters such as Rembrandt, Dürer and Fragonard, the satirical drawings and pictures of Rowlandson and Hogarth, a variety of Victorian painters, Picasso, Freud and Hockney, to name only a few who could have been included. We hope you will enjoy our final selection.

This ABC is intended to be an update, and a summary of a wide range of sexual matters and will, I hope, be a help to those who want to be more informed about what is actually going on in the world. If the contributors to this series have enabled colleagues of whatever discipline to be more knowledgeable and relaxed about sexual matters, they will be well pleased.

1. Weston JAB and Tomlinson JM. The Guildford (University of Surrey) release course for trainee general practitioners. *J R Coll Gen Pract* 1984;**34**:82–86.
2. Ray, C. *Sex education*. Highlight series No. 168, Sex Education Forum, National Children's Bureau, London 1999.
3. Wiltshire C. *The Times* 1999, February 27

Acknowledgements

My thanks are due to Richard Smith, the Editor of the BMJ, who encouraged the Editorial Board to published this series in the Journal, as well as to Greg Cotton, Technical Editor and Jan Croot, Pictures Editor for their patience and help at all times. I am particularly grateful to all those correspondents who, personally, by e-mail or by letter welcomed the series so warmly, and I hope that any errors have been corrected.

John Tomlinson

1 Management of sexual problems

Margaret Ramage

Sexual problems present in various ways, many indirect or covert. Patients do not like to come straight to the point. They fear looking stupid by using wrong words, or giving offence by being too explicit, or they have no way of conceptualising what it is that is wrong. A doctor can find himself or herself fumbling around in a slightly mad conversation in which nobody understands what is being said. A common language needs to be established first, particularly in sexual medicine, followed by a good history and a careful examination, if appropriate, before an assessment of relevant management can be made. Recurrent gynaecological or urological complaints, insomnia, depression, joint pains, and other symptoms have all been used as covert presentations of sexual problems.

Once the presence of a sexual problem has been established, its severity and importance to the patient need to be understood before the most appropriate course of management can be offered. This can vary from straightforward education, by simply giving accurate information, to referral for psychiatric assessment (fortunately very rare). History taking is therefore the paramount skill underpinning decisions about management, along with forming a positive alliance with the patient. Any course of action has to have complete cooperation. Without that, the best treatment in the world may be useless.

Overall management

It is worth bearing in mind that, however obviously physical the cause of a sexual problem, there may well be psychological sequelae, if not for the patient then for his or her partner if there is one. Conversely, when the cause seems to be entirely psychological there may be hidden organic factors at work, and it would be irresponsible to miss them. Thus overall management has to take account of both aspects (exclusion of organic factors is covered later in the series).

Psychological approaches

Giving accurate information
It is useful to give accurate and relevant information. Various books and videos are available that patients may find helpful.

Some sexual problems can be solved with an in vivo anatomy lesson, especially if the patient lacks a knowledge of the basics of sexual anatomy and physiology and the normal changes of ageing. It can be particularly invaluable to a woman who has never examined herself or to a man worried about the size of his genitals.

The sexual arousal circuit
A challenge to clinicians is to enable patients to understand that sexual problems happen in response to something and are not usually located solely in the genitals. Relationships, early learning about sex, trauma, and life stresses can all contribute. A diagram of the sexual arousal circuit is beneficial to show how these factors may all be linked to a sexual problem.[1] When explained to patients, it can help them understand the possible roots of their problem, and thus the appropriate choices for its management.

At its simplest, sexual arousal is a straightforward spinal reflex triggered by appropriate stimulation of the body,

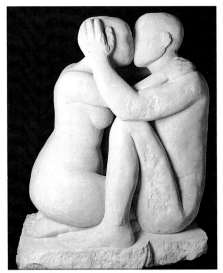

Man, Woman and Fish by Emily Young

Useful guides

Videos
The mature couple's guide to love and intimacy. In the series *Sex, a lifelong pleasure.* London: Visual Corporation (tel: 01371 873 138)

Lovers' guide (a series introduced by Dr Andrew Stanway). London: Carlton Home Entertainment (tel: 0181 207 6207)

Books
Zilbergeld B. *Men and sex: a guide to sexual fulfilment.* London: Fontana, 1986

Brown P, Faulder C. *Treat yourself to sex.* London: Penguin, 1989

Litvinoff S. *Relate guide to loving relationships.* London: Ebury Press, 1992

Eid JF, Pearce CA. *Making love again. Regaining sexual potency through the new injection treatment.* New York: Brunner Maazel, 1993

Quilliam S. *Your sexual self.* London: Cassell, 1997

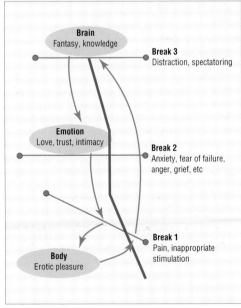

The sexual arousal circuit, a schematic representation of the factors that can positively or negatively affect the sexual response in the body, the mind, and the emotions

often, but not necessarily, the genital area. This is interpreted in the brain and moderated by the emotions, so that events in those two arenas will exert a powerful influence over that reflex. Sexual response can be described as an electrical circuit that can start anywhere—mind, body, or emotion—but which also has three break points, one in each area.

The first break point occurs when there is inappropriate stimulation or pain. Pain can automatically cancel any possibility of response. Common problems are inappropriate stimulation of the clitoris and, in particular, insufficient stimulation of the penis as men get older, a point not widely appreciated.

The second break point (and probably the most powerful) occurs in the emotional arena, and a patient can be paralysed by fear of failure, anxiety, and pressure to perform. Other negative emotions important in this context include anger, unresolved conflict (in any area of life), undisclosed resentment, and grief.

The third break point occurs when the mind is too busy for the individual to relax and become aroused. An example of this, common in men with erectile dysfunction, is "spectatoring," when the mind is focused on observing the performance of the penis to the exclusion of almost everything else. Others include distraction caused by worries about work, memories of negative experiences, expectations of failure, and uncertainty of how to behave.

General counselling

Counselling can uncover and help resolve hidden conflicts or the emotions of anger and grief long denied. Any issues about relationships may also be explored in this context, and communication between partners, often difficult in the presence of sexual problems, can be facilitated. An environment of emotional support and understanding can help patients work out their own solutions, with establishment of realistic goals and support for any changes in lifestyle.

Psychosexual therapy

The assumption underlying this therapy is that the relationship between therapist and patient provides a mirror of the relationship the patient has with his or her partner. It enables understanding of any disturbed interaction with the partner and any hidden conflicts in the patient. Initially, the doctor asks questions only when necessary, to minimise leading the patient. Medical investigations and questioning can sometimes be a way of avoiding painful and important emotional matters that the patient or the doctor may be afraid to face.

It is most important to be aware of the feelings evoked in the doctor as well as the patient as the patient's story unfolds and the physical examination takes place. These feelings need to be discussed with the patient and can be used to inform him or her of the inner conflicts causing the difficulties. Treatment is tailored to a patient's individual needs to enable an understanding of the unique unconscious blocks hindering sexual fulfilment.

This technique has been developed to be useful in a relatively short interview and so does not necessarily require any commitment to regular therapy sessions. Many general practitioners and some practice nurses have been trained in this approach, which lends itself well to the setting of a general practice or family planning clinic.

Behavioural approach

A man with premature ejaculation can learn to delay his ejaculation by means of a programme of graded masturbatory exercises (the squeeze technique), with or

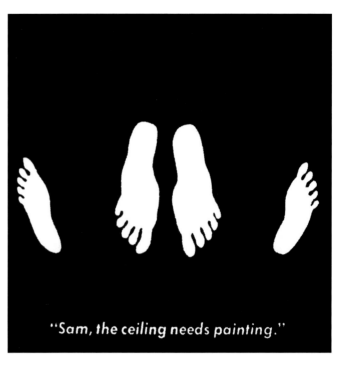

"Sam, the ceiling needs painting."

The third break point in the sexual arousal circuit occurs when the mind is too busy for the individual to relax and become aroused

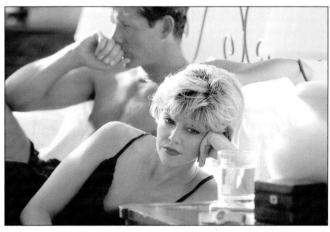

Counselling can uncover and help resolve hidden conflicts or long denied anger and grief

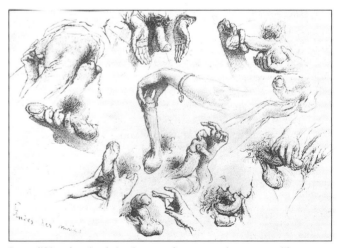

By modifying the stimulation in masturbatory exercises, a man with premature ejaculation can learn to slow his response. (Studies of masturbation from *Love* (1911) by Mihaly von Zichy)

without drug treatment. The aim of the exercises is to enable the patient to recognise the feelings in his penis at different levels of arousal and, by modifying the stimulation, to learn to slow his response.

Vaginismus can also be dealt with behaviourally (see later article in this series). Patients with compulsive sexual behaviour or paraphilia are likely to be most effectively treated with a programme of behaviour modification under supervision (see later article). The behavioural approach would not ordinarily address any underlying psychological factors, but this is not always so.

Sexual and relationship therapy

This integrated therapy incorporates psychodynamic, behavioural, cognitive, and systemic principles. The relationship may be viewed as "the patient," rather than either partner as an individual. After thorough assessment of physical, psychological, and, particularly if a couple comes together, relationship factors, a therapeutic contract is made, with clearly stated goals if possible and sometimes a limited number of sessions. The patient or couple may agree to homework tasks to facilitate and maintain changes. Family influences and cultural and gender issues may also be seen as important, and communication between partners is often fundamental in this approach. With a sexual problem, the relationship will inevitably be affected, but this can commonly offer the very vehicle to ameliorate the situation.

Once communication between partners is open and constructive, therapeutic tasks can be assigned to them to enable them to resolve their difficulties in the privacy of their own home and at times to suit their lifestyle. It is the job of the therapist to work out with them what would be most helpful. The feedback from these tasks, together with the appropriate management of any important emotional material arising from them, provides the route whereby many sexual problems can be resolved.

Sensate focus

This is a programme of tasks, first described by Masters and Johnson in 1970,[2] that a couple can undertake in their own time at home. Underlying the programme is a ban on sexual intercourse or any genital contact until anxiety about performance and fear of failure have subsided and trust between the couple has been established. This ban ensures that physical intimacy will not lead to sexual intimacy. The tasks involve the couple setting aside time to explore each other's bodies in turn by touching, stroking, caressing, and massaging— gradually introducing sensual, then erotic, and then sexual touch over a period of time.

The couple need to be monitored, to agree the ground rules and the staged tasks, to deal with any issues that may arise as a result of the tasks, to support positive changes and prevent relapse in the early stages.

Suggested ground rules are
- Agree a ban on sexual intercourse and genital touching
- Set up twice weekly times to spend on this homework, increasing from 20 minutes to 60 minutes over 4 weeks
- During these times, speak only if the partner's touch is painful or unacceptable. Otherwise it is assumed that what is being done is all right. Conversation will prevent concentration on the task and render it pointless
- Attention should be focused on personal experience, not on pleasing the partner
- This is a learning exercise above all

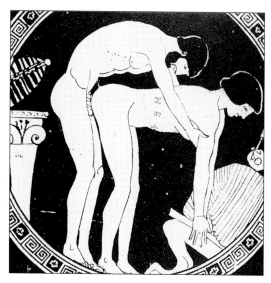

Partners can be assigned tasks to enable them to resolve their difficulties in the privacy of their own home (Athenian cup painting by Douris, 500-460 BC)

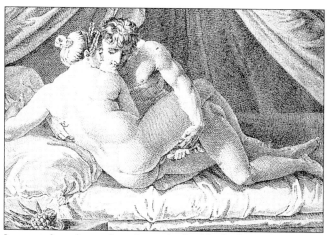

In sensate focus the couple explore each other's bodies by touching, stroking, and caressing. (*Antoine et Cleopatre* (c. 1602) by Agostino Carracci)

Sensate focus

Stage 1
1—Taking plenty of time, each person explores the other's naked (if possible) body, avoiding breasts and genitals, avoiding trying to give pleasure, and concentrating on feelings and sensations experienced in both "active" and "passive" roles
2—After 2 weeks or 4 sessions of this, some familiarity and trust should allow inclusion of breasts and experimentation with a variety of touches, such as with body oils, talcum powder, feathers, fabrics, etc
3—As above but adding the making of specific requests for preferred types of touch and the use of a back to front position to enable the person being touched to guide the partner's hand

Stage 2
1—Maintain the ban on intercourse, but include genital touching as part of the established exercises, so there are now no forbidden areas
2—While continuing all the above, concentrate more on the genitals to discover the sensations resulting from different pressures in different areas
3—This is an optional stage for mutual masturbation to orgasm

Stage 3
1—While continuing all the above and maintaining the ban on full intercourse, the next step is containment without movement, allowing the penis to be accepted and contained by the vagina (modified for homosexual couples). Couples should progress at their preferred pace
2—Containment with gentle thrusting and rotating movement
3—Thrusting to orgasm

Physical remedies

Pharmacological and surgical treatment will be covered in later articles.

Lubricants—KY Jelly and Senselle are generally well tolerated by both men and women and are available in high street stores. Carrier oils as used in aromatherapy, such as peach kernel and sweet almond oils, can be an excellent substitute for those who find water based lubricants are an irritant or messy (but must not be used with latex contraceptives, as the oil rots the rubber very rapidly, making them ineffective).

Tension rings—These are useful when an adequate erection can be obtained but not sustained. A tight rubber band at the base of the penis maintains an erection for up to 30 minutes.

Vacuum pumps—These promote an erection, which a tension ring can then sustain. Pumps are available in both battery and manual forms.

Vibrators—These are available from sex shops and catalogues. The Clairol Heat Massager is obtainable from high street stores and has the advantage of being useful in other contexts. It is mains operated, which may be a further advantage.

Use of surrogates

Masters and Johnson used surrogate partners for patients who presented with sexual dysfunction but who had no partner, and Cole has described the use of surrogates in Britain.[3] With a surrogate, a man might gain a sexual confidence that he could take into another relationship, but all relationships have their own chemistry and dynamic, and the erection might well not be portable. The practice was later abandoned by these workers, as complex legal, contractual, and ethical issues are raised. For example, where would responsibility lie if a patient were or became infected with HIV?

Referral onwards

Most patients with sexual problems expect to be referred on or at least investigated medically. It is very useful if the referrer has some personal knowledge or contact with the next clinician.

A list of therapists can be obtained from the Institute of Psychosexual Medicine (11 Chandos Street, London W1M 9DE) who also train doctors in the practical skills of psychosexual medicine, or the British Association for Sexual and Marital Therapy (PO Box 13686, London SW20 9HZ). Relate-Marriage Guidance also gives further specialised training in sexual therapy (a list of local centres can be obtained from its office at Herbert Gray College, Little Church Street, Rugby CV21 3AP).

The picture of *Man, Woman and Fish* is reproduced with permission of Emily Young, courtesy of the Thackeray Gallery, London (private collection). The cartoon "Sam, the ceiling needs painting" is by Neville Spearman. The photograph of the couple lying in bed is reproduced with permission of Tony Stone. The engraving by Zichy is reproduced with permission of the Bridgeman Art Library Stapleton Collection.

1 Stanley E. Principles of managing sexual problems. *BMJ* 1981;282:1200-2.
2 Masters WH, Johnson VE. *Human sexual inadequacy.* London: Churchill, 1970.
3 Cole M. Sex therapy for individuals. In: Cole M, Dryden W, eds. *Sex therapy in Britain.* Milton Keynes: Open University Press, 1988.

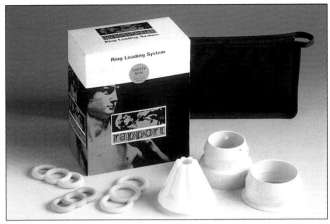

Tension rings can maintain an erection for up to 30 minutes when placed at the base of the penis

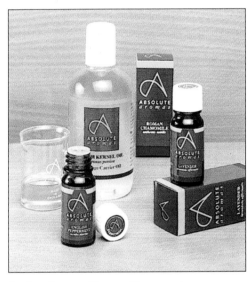

Carrier oils, as used in aromatherapy and massage, can be used as an alternative to water based lubricants for facilitating sexual intercourse

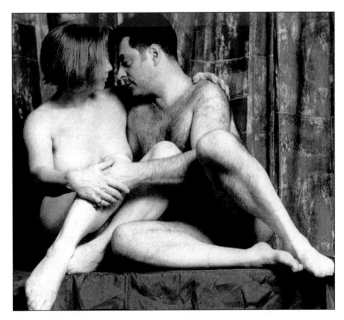

With a surrogate partner, a man might gain sexual confidence. (Picture reproduced with subjects' written permission)

2 Normal male anatomy, physiology, and behaviour

John Tomlinson

Many adult men (and a large number of women) are ignorant of the structure and function of the male sexual organs, although the penis is used for micturition and boys become accustomed to handling their genitalia from an early age. It is important to be clear on their structure and function (see later chapter for anatomy and physiology of sexual function by Kirby) to clarify misapprehensions and myths.

Anatomy and physiology

The penis

This consists of two parallel corpora cavernosa (cavernous bodies) in line with the corpus spongiosum (spongy body), which encircles the urethra on the underside of the penis and expands at its tip to form the glans. Proximally, the corpora cavernosa are attached to the pelvis just anterior to the ischial tuberosities, and binding the three together is a thick fascia, Buck's fascia, covered in turn by the superficial or Colles fascia. The trabecular structure of the corpora consists of smooth muscle and fibroelastic tissue; the muscle relaxes on sexual arousal, causing the penis to become erect with incoming blood. Over all this is the very loose and mobile penile skin, which allows the penis to expand during erection

The glans—The glans, which surrounds the urethral meatus, consists entirely of corpus spongiosum and has a large concentration of sensory nerve endings from the pudendal nerves, particularly round the coronal rim and underneath at the frenulum, the thin fold of skin which attaches the glans to the foreskin.

The foreskin—In most uncircumcised men the glans pushes out to a varying extent from the encircling foreskin during sexual arousal. In a small proportion of young men the frenulum is tight, which may cause bowing of the end of the penis on erection or even difficulty in retracting the foreskin. Generally, it stretches in use, but it sometimes rips during intercourse, with much bleeding and anguish for the man and his partner. If the frenulum causes problems it can easily be snipped in a general practitioner's treatment room.

Circumcision—In a recent large survey in the United Kingdom 21.9% of all men, including Jews and Muslims, had been circumcised, but this varied with age.[1] Only 12.5% of men aged 16–24 were circumcised compared with 32.3% of those aged 45–59, probably a reflection of changing public health policies from the 1940s.

As the penis varies markedly in appearance from one man to another—in colour, length, girth, shape, and presence of a foreskin—its size and shape can cause a considerable amount of worry to its owner. The length of the flaccid penis is 5–9.5 cm. The erect penis varies much less in size than is generally believed, and the normal range is 12.5–17.5 cm,[2] with an average of 16 cm, and a distal girth (measured just proximal to the glans) averaging 12 cm.

Anxiety about size is perpetuated by men not realising that a smaller penis enlarges by a greater percentage volume than a larger flaccid penis, that magazine photographs are carefully angled, that especially well endowed "actors" or models are chosen for videos, and, importantly, that when a

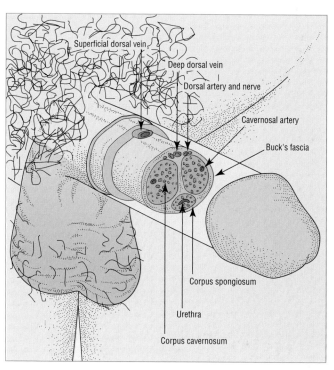

Diagram of anatomy of the penis. Adapted from *Impotence* by Foster MC and Cole M with permission of Schwarz Pharma.

Uncircumcising*

A doctor who had been circumcised as a child had had minor discomfort in his glans for years, always having to wear tight underwear. He noticed that there was remarkably little sensitivity in the glans but assumed that little could be done about it until he read a book on uncircumcising (J Bigelow's *The Joy of Uncircumcising!* Hourglass Books, 1992).

He decided to refashion his foreskin and stretched the penile skin with weights and surgical tape. By 10 days, he was more comfortable than he had ever been, and, after 10 weeks, intercourse was easier and frictionless. He continued and was delighted, and concluded that doctors and medical students need to be taught that the foreskin has function and is as important to the penis as the eyelid to the eye—a protector, moistener, and sensitiser—and he advocated conservatism, especially in treating phimosis.

* Story taken from Personal view: The joy of uncircumcising. *BMJ* 1994;309:676-7

> **An 80 year old man, on being given a test dose of alprostadil for erectile dysfunction, was delighted on being told that his feeling of shame at his small penis for the past 65 years was completely unjustified and that his size was well within the normal range**

man looksdown he sees a foreshortened view of himself. Erections larger than 20 cm in white men are unusual, and claims have to be taken with a pinch of salt.[2]

The scrotum

This varies in external appearance under different circumstances. In young people, in cold weather, with exercise, and during the excitement and plateau phases of sexual stimulation the subcutaneous dartos muscle contracts and the scrotal skin is corrugated and closely applied to the testes. In warmth, under loose clothing, and in older men the scrotum hangs elongated and flaccid, allowing a fall in temperature of up to 1.0°C, believed to enhance sperm production.

The testes

The testes measure about 5×2.5×2.5 cm but can vary in size from day to day in the same person, and with the left usually hanging lower than the right. Production of spermatozoa and testosterone are under the control of the hypothalamus, which produces gonadotrophin releasing hormone (GnRH), which in turn controls the pituitary's release of luteinising hormone (LH), responsible for production of testosterone, and follicle stimulating hormone (FSH), which stimulates production of spermatozoa and oestrogen.

Spermatozoa travel from the seminiferous tubules to the seminal vesicles, where up to 70% of the total ejaculate is formed, the rest coming from the prostate, which is the first to be ejaculated and which contains the highest concentration of sperms. Although the seminal vesicles are said not to store sperms, despite their name, no one has clearly identified where the sperms that are found in the first 10-20 ejaculates after vasectomy are stored.

Semen is usually thick and sticky immediately after ejaculation but rapidly liquefies, leading some patients to think erroneously that the quality of their sperm has diminished or become "thin."

Cowper's glands—These two subprostatic, paraurethral, pea sized glands produce a clear, slightly sticky fluid at the penile meatus on sexual arousal. This varies in quantity from a bead to 5 ml, although some men are not aware of it at all. Colloquially known as pre-come (or pre-cum), it seems to be a natural lubricant and may contain a few live spermatozoa.

The breasts

Men have only a very small amount of breast tissue, but at puberty one or other breast may enlarge and become painful, causing acute embarrassment to the adolescent. This gynaecomastia usually settles within a year or so, but, rarely, it may be severe enough to warrant a breast reduction. Carcinoma of the adult male breast can occur but is uncommon, occurring in about 1 in 1200 men.

Other erogenous zones

These include the mouth, skin, and the anus and rectum. The anus is highly sensitive, and insertion of a finger or other object (including a penis) is not uncommon in heterosexual as well as homosexual intercourse. In a survey of US men aged 20–39, 20% claimed to have taken part in anal intercourse at least once, although only 2% of them had had penetrative sex with another man.[3]

Puberty

The anatomical and physiological changes of puberty occur one to two years later than in girls, with an adolescent growth spurt on average at 14 years. The earliest change is in

---

> A 20 year old undergraduate, after enjoying his first sexual encounter, was mortified and humiliated the next day to hear that his partner had told all his friends (male and female) how small and poorly endowed he was genitally. He became completely impotent until he was seen in an erectile dysfunction clinic. After treatment with alprostadil, he was shown with a tape measure that he was actually at the upper level of the normal range of length and girth. He recovered full function

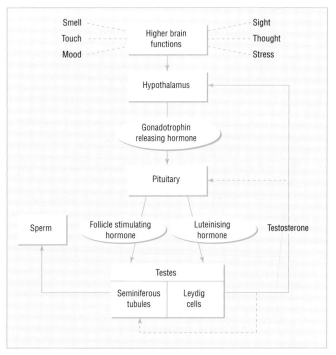

Endocrine regulation of sperm production

Assessing endocrine function

- A low serum testosterone concentration often leads to reduced sexual interest and erectile dysfunction, but many men can perform normally
- Serum testosterone concentration alone is not a reliable guide
- The biologically available testosterone, the free androgen index (FAI), is a better guide and is found by dividing the testosterone concentration by the serum hormone binding globulin (SHBG) concentration, expressed as a percentage
- Most authorities would treat with replacement testosterone if the free androgen index is much below 50%, although a level down to 35% is accepted by many as still normal.
- It is essential to try and exclude a carcinoma of the prostrate before giving replacement testosterone. Digital rectal examination and a serum prostatic specific antigen (PSA) should be done in all prospective recipients.
- A high luteinising hormone (LH) concentration suggests that the interstitial, or Leydig, cells, which manufacture testosterone are not responding
- A low luteinising hormone concentration may indicate that the pituitary is not producing enough

the growth of the testes as a result of luteinising hormone stimulating testosterone production. As this increases, so the penis, prostate, and seminal vesicles grow. As soon as sufficient testosterone is present for them to function, ejaculation is possible.

Sperm production starts in childhood and becomes fully established when or soon after ejaculation is possible. Boys begin to undergo genital development at an average age of 11.6 years, with the genitals reaching adult size and shape by an average of 14.9 years. Some boys develop rapidly over a year while others can take up to five years.[4] The youngest recorded father of a child in Britain in modern times was an 11 year old boy in 1997 who claimed to have made a 14 year old girl pregnant. A healthy baby was born in January 1998.[5]

Nocturnal and early morning rections are a normal part of paradoxical or REM sleep (and are not connected with having a full bladder). A 13 year old will have, on average, four erections a night and, for about a third of his time sleeping, has penile tumescence. This rate falls slowly to two or more erections occupying a fifth of sleeping time in men in their 60s.[6] Nocturnal emissions ("wet dreams") seem to be a physiological safety valve, occurring in over 80% of men at some time, with two thirds of 17 year olds having at least one a month. There is then a rapid decline so that few over the age of 30 continue.

Masturbation is now seen as a healthy form of sexual expression and is fortunately no longer regarded as dirty and sinful, as it used to be when religious authority saw it as a threat to health and morality. It has been estimated that 95% of men have masturbated, and frequency seems to vary from daily to once a month, with the highest incidence in the teens and early 20s, and very much depends on other sexual activities.[7]

Hair starts to develop on the pubis with the start of genital growth, with axillary hair following some 12–24 months later. Chest hair growth may start during puberty or later and may continue growing for 10 or more years. Deepening of the voice is caused by testosterone stimulation of the larynx, which lengthens anteriorly. The average age of voice change is now 13.5 years, compared with 18 years in 1750.[8]

Sexual intercourse

The proportion of boys in Britain who experience sexual intercourse before the age of 16 has increased to a sizeable minority—27.6% in 1994[1]—although the median age rises with the level of education and with those from the Indian subcontinent, but a much larger proportion of black youths than white start intercourse before the age of 16. The main factors that tempt boys to start include spur of the moment action (44.2%) and curiosity (40.5%).

Sexual arousal and response

Masters and Johnson discovered the four stages of sexual response in men.[7] Most information comes from their work in the 1960s and 1970s, and they parallel those in women.

Stage 1: excitement phase

This results from physical or psychological stimulation, or both, which can rapidly lead to erection of the penis and drawing up of the testes (for detailed pharmacology of the response, see later chapter). The corpora fill with blood from the helicine arteries via the internal iliac and pudendal arteries. Tiredness and anxiety can interfere with this seemingly simple procedure, and a man's erection may not be solidly firm despite his being aroused. At detumescence, the blood drains via the deep dorsal, cavernosal, and crural veins.

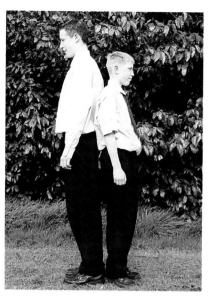

Two boys aged 14·3 developing at different rates (180 and 165 cm)

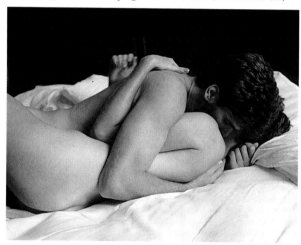

The main factors that tempt boys are spur of the moment action and curiosity

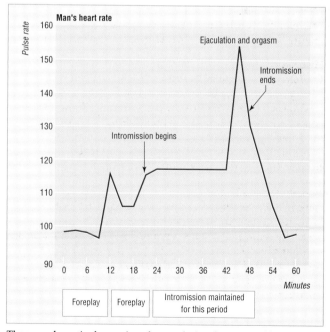

There are dramatic changes in pulse-rate during the course of human copulatory activities. During foreplay the male pulse-rate slowly increases; then, with intromission, it reaches a high plateau level and finally peaks at around 150 with ejaculation. (Adapted from Morris D. *Manwatching*. Triad Granada, 1978)

Stage 2: plateau stage

The diameter of the glans increases and deepens in colour with vasocongestion, which also causes the testes to become up to 50% larger. The testes continue to rise, and there is a feeling of perineal warmth. The buttocks and thighs tighten, the heart rate increases, respiration is quicker, and blood pressure rises slightly. Orgasm is imminent.

Stage 3: orgasm and ejaculation

These are different processes which can be selectively impaired, but they are generally taken to be synonymous (colloquially called "climax" or "coming"). The vas deferens, prostate, and seminal vesicles begin a series of contractions that force semen into the bulb of the urethra—the so called brink of control, when ejaculation cannot be stopped—and then contractions of the prostate and urethra lead to ejaculation. The rectal sphincter and the neck of the bladder tighten while the contractions force the semen out. Orgasms vary at different times in the same person and from person to person, depending on circumstances—mood, partner, occasion, frequency.

Stage 4: resolution

After ejaculation there is a refractory or recovery time, when further orgasm is not possible. A partial or even full erection may sometimes be maintained during this period, especially in younger men. Recovery time varies from a few minutes to many hours, or even a couple of days in elderly men. Detumescence now occurs, and the changes of stage 1 reverse, with the addition of heavy fast respiration, a tachycardia, and sometimes profuse sweating. Sexual arousal without orgasm can lead to resolution being slower, with a pelvic fullness and penile and testicular aching of varying intensity due to vasocongestion.

The effects of age

Sexual ability and drive continue well into old age, although there is a decline in frequency of activity. This can be partially explained by poorer health, but it is also partly due to cultural expectations.

Compared with younger men, men aged over 55 usually take a longer time and require more direct manual or oral stimulation for the penis to become erect, tend to have less firm erections, produce a smaller amount of semen and have a less intense ejaculation. They usually have less physical need to ejaculate, and have a longer refractory period and reduced muscle tension.[7]

An older man with erectile dysfunction is often humiliated and demoralised to be told by his doctor, "What can you expect at your age?" and fear of this dissuades many from asking for help. In a survey of elderly in 1988, 62% of the men aged between 80 and 102 were still having sexual intercourse.[7] The importance attached to regular intercourse in younger days correlated significantly with sexual activity in old age. The adage "If you don't use it, you lose it" has more than a grain of truth. There is obviously no reason to deny that men (and women) can enjoy sexual activity to a ripe old age.

The figure of endocrine regulation of sperm production is adapted from Masters WH, John VE, Kolodny RC. *Human sexuality.* 5th ed. New York: Harper Collins, 1995. The figure of the sexual response cycle in men is adapted from Masters WH, Johnson VE. *Human sexual response.* Boston MA: Little, Brown, 1966. All figures are used with the publishers' permission. The painting by Botticelli is reproduced with permission of Bridgeman Art Library. The photograph of the two boys is reproduced with their and their parents' permission. The cartoon "You can still manage it..." is reproduced with permission of Tony Goffe.

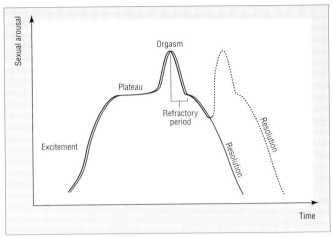

The sexual response cycle in men. Dotted line shows possibility of second orgasm and ejaculation after the refractory period. (Redrawn from Master WH, Johnson VE. *Human Sexual Response.* Boston, MA: Little, Brown, 1966)

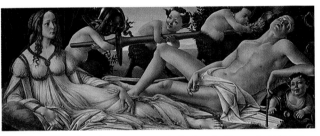

After ejacualtion there is a recovery period, when further orgasm is not possible. (*Venus and Mars*, circa, Sandro Botticelli)

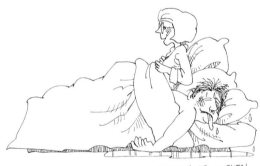

" WELL DEAR, YOU CAN STILL MANAGE IT — EVEN AT YOUR AGE ....."

1 Johnson AM, Wadsworth J, Wellings K, Field F. *Sexual attitudes and lifestyles.* Oxford: Blackwell Scientific, 1994
2 Dickinson RL. *Human sex anatomy.* London: Kreiger Publishing, 1971. In Coxon APM. *Between the sheets: project SIGMA.* London: Cassell, 1996
3 Billy JOG, Tanfer K, Grady WR, Klepinger DH.. The sexual behaviour of men in the United States. *Family Planning Perspectives* 1993;25:52-60
4 Marshall WA, Tanner JM. Variation in the pubertal changes in boys. *Arch Dis Child* 1970;45:13-23
5 *Daily Telegraph* 1998 Jan 21
6 Bancroft J. *Human sexuality and its problems.* 2nd ed. Edinburgh: Churchill Livingstone, 1989
7 Masters WH, Johnson VE, Kolodny RC. *Human sexuality.* 5th ed. New York: Harper Collins, 1995
8 Grumbach M. The neuroendocrinology of puberty. *Hosp Pract* 1980 Mar:51-60
9 Bretschneider JG, McCoy NL. Sexual interest and behaviour in healthy 80-102 year olds. *Arch Sex Behav* 1988;17:109-27

3 Normal female sexual anatomy, physiology, and behaviour

Tony Parsons

Puberty

Functional adult sexual anatomy and physiology are established during the course of puberty. This process, which is spread over several years, consists of a series of overlapping developments including growth and development of the breasts, growth of pubic and axillary hair, accelerated growth in height, and, finally, menstruation and ovulation. The age at which each stage is reached varies widely, such that one girl may have completed the process at an age when another has not even started.

Early menstrual cycles are usually irregular, and ovulation may take one to two years to be established after the first period. During this time, the womb lining is being built up and shed in response to changes in oestrogen levels only. Once ovulation begins, the production of progesterone in the corpus luteum controls the timing of the cycles, but this also triggers the process which leads to dysmenorrhoea.

Although there has been a gradual trend for menarche to occur at a younger age during this century, this only partially explains the reduction in age at first sexual experience and first sexual intercourse. A recent British survey found that 18.7% of women had started intercourse before the age of 16 (compared with 27.6% of men),[1] whereas 40 years ago it was fewer than 1%.

Sexual anatomy

The external genitalia, or vulva, consist of the mons veneris, the labia, the clitoris, and the perineum. All are heavily innervated with sensory nerve fibres and are involved in the physiological processes of sexual response. The mons veneris is particularly sensitive to touch or pressure sensation. The labia are an important source of sexual sensation for most women, and the labia minora have a spongy core, which become engorged on arousal. The clitoris consists of the clitoral glans and shaft, which are covered by the clitoral hood. The clitoris itself is highly sensitive to touch, pressure, and temperature and is subject to indirect stimulation during intercourse by the movement of the labia minora. Bartholin's glands, which lie posteriorly within the labia minora, were thought to be responsible for vaginal lubrication, but they are now considered of minor importance.

Many people, especially men, do not realise that the vagina has few sensory nerve endings except at the introitus, and, therefore, the inner two thirds of the vagina are relatively insensitive. In a non-parous woman, the average lengths of the posterior and anterior walls are 7.5 cm and 6 cm respectively. The concept of the G (Grafenburg) spot, a particularly sensitive region in the front wall of the vagina midway between the pubic bone and the cervix,[2] remains controversial and has not been proved scientifically. The cervix itself is highly variable in its sensitivity and often plays no role in sexual enjoyment.

Many other parts of the body as well as those involved in reproduction are potential sources of sexual arousal. The insides of the thigh, the neck, and the perineum are often erogenous zones, as is the mouth, including the lips and the tongue. The anal canal and perianal area are also highly sensitive to touch, and anal stimulation or intercourse can be part of normal heterosexual activity.

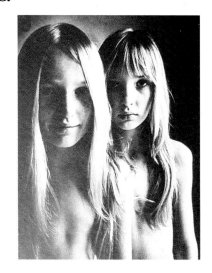

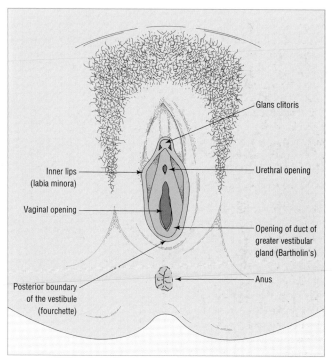

Female genitalia with labia parted. Redrawn from Banfield J. Human sexuality and its problems, 2nd edn. Edinburgh: Churchill Livingstone, 1989

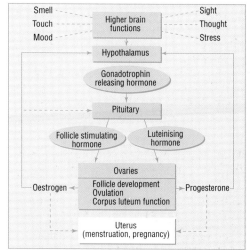

Endocrine regulation of sexual development in women

Physiology of sexual response

A physiological sexual response requires intact pelvic innervation, adequate local blood supply, and a normal hormonal environment. Sexual arousal can occur under a wide variety of situations and may be triggered purely by cerebral events or by response to physical contact. Excitement, however, is not invariably linked to arousal. It is possible for women under some circumstances to show the physiological changes of arousal without experiencing any of the pleasurable sensations normally associated with this. Episodes of vaginal lubrication also occur during sleep (in the same way as nocturnal erections) and are not controlled by the specific content of dreams.

Our understanding of the sexual response cycle is based largely on the original observations of Masters and Johnson[3] and assumes that their sample of volunteer subjects was representative of the full range of normal physiology. Their classification divides sexual response into four phases: excitement, plateau, orgasm, and resolution. The phases represent an incremental increase in sexual excitement, and each is a necessary precursor for the next phase. It has been suggested that an extra phase normally precedes these—the desire phase, the part of sexual response that is perhaps the least understood.

Excitement or arousal phase

This is the initial response to sexual stimulation and, like each phase, has both genital and systemic components. The reflex of vasodilatation within the genitalia is mediated through two centres in the spinal cord (one at the level T1l-L2, the other at S2–S4) and through specific receptors in the pelvic smooth muscle. Increased blood flow in the vaginal wall results in a transudate through the vaginal walls, which is the main source of lubrication. At the same time the inner two thirds of the vagina balloon out or "tent," and the vulva becomes engorged.

The systemic component of this phase includes increases in pulse and respiratory rates and blood pressure. Some women also show general vasocongestion, especially over the upper torso and neck. The excitement phase is vulnerable to interruption by distraction, internally such as by extraneous thoughts or by interruption.

Plateau phase

This is sometimes regarded as part of arousal and represents a consolidation of the changes that occurred during the excitement phase. Congestion in the outer third of the vagina reaches a maximum, producing a firm area of engorged tissue around the introitus (the so called "orgasmic platform"). Breast changes also reach a maximum in this phase: breast size may increase by 20–25% in many women who have not breast fed, and the areolae become congested so that the nipple looks less erect. Finally, as orgasm approaches, the clitoris becomes firmly retracted against the pubic bone and seems to disappear. Although described as a plateau, this phase actually requires continuous stimulation to build up sexual excitement to the intensity that is necessary for orgasm.

Orgasm

Objectively, orgasm is a peak of pleasurable sensation and the release of the sexual tension that has built up during the preceding phases, together with involuntary rhythmic contraction of the genital muscles (at 0.8 second intervals).

Subjectively, orgasms differ widely in their description from one woman to another and from one occasion to another, although descriptions of orgasm by men and by

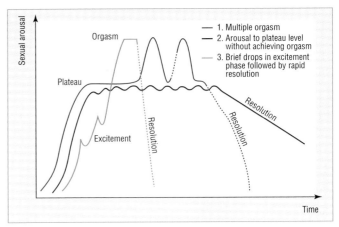

Sexual response cycle in women. (Redrawn from Masters WH, Johnson VE. *Human Sexual Response.* Boston MA: Little Brown, 1996.)

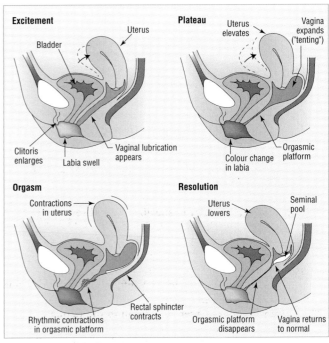

Internal changes occurring in female sexual response

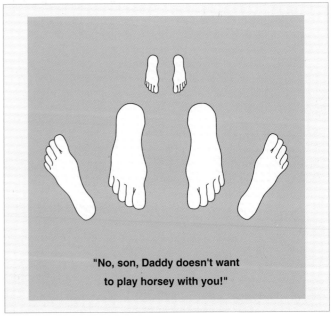

"No, son, Daddy doesn't want to play horsey with you!"

The excitement phase is vulnerable to interruption by distraction women are remarkably similar. The importance of orgasm for sexual satisfaction may also vary. After orgasm, most women do not have the refractory period that is seen in men, and further stimulation can produce further orgasms.

It is clear that the nature of the orgasm is not affected by the type of stimulation used to produce it, although masturbatory orgasms may be somewhat more intense. Many men do not realise that fewer than one in three women can reach a climax from coitus alone and that foreplay, such as stimulation of the clitoris (manually or orally) and touching and caressing other erogenous zones, is essential for orgasm to occur in the majority.

Resolution

After orgasm, the body gradually returns to the non-aroused state. In older, parous women impairment of this resolution phase, especially if associated with high levels of arousal and failure to climax, may lead to pelvic congestion with non-specific symptoms of aching in the lower back and pelvis, which has its exact counterpart in men.

Menopause

The menopause may have an impact on women's sexuality in three main ways.

Psychologically, it may represent a watershed and a point beyond which a woman feels she no longer can, or should, be sexually attractive.

Physical symptoms, particularly severe night sweats and mood swings, can be highly disruptive to a sexual relationship.

Oestrogen deficiency causes specific physical responses in some women. These include a failure of vaginal lubrication (this may start before the actual cessation of periods), development of vaginal dryness and irritation, reduced sensation in the vulval tissues, and impaired neural transmission of these sensations. Painful uterine contractions at orgasm seem to be more common after the menopause. The natural loss of collagen may result in the vagina becoming less elastic, particularly in those who are not sexually active. The vaginal introitus and the surrounding vulva may atrophy. Long term oestrogen replacement (either systemically or as a cream locally) may be needed to prevent or reverse these changes.

Sexual drive

Sexual drive is clearly complex but poorly understood. There is probably a hormonal element underlying both sexual interest and the ability to respond, but there are no clear patterns. There is considerable variation from one woman to another, particularly during the menstrual cycle and pregnancy. Studies have shown that women who have a less satisfactory sexual life or who are unable to discuss their sexuality openly with their partner are most likely to experience a reduction in sexual satisfaction when they pass through a time of physiological change. Sexual drive may actually improve at the menopause, but when it is reduced (either as a primary problem or because of vaginal dryness) oestrogen replacement is often highly effective.

Although there is a general tendency for sexual drive to decrease with age (and duration of relationship), there are no upper age limits for a happy active sexual life.

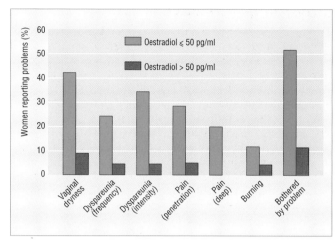

Effect of serum oestradiol concentrations on reported sexual problems in postmenopausal women. (Adapted from Sarrel P. Sexuality and menopause. *J Obstet Gynaecol* 1990;75: 265-355)

Symptoms associated with urogenital ageing

- Vaginal dryness
- Vaginal irritation
- Dyspareunia
- Postcoital bleeding
- Urinary frequency and urgency

Effects of oestrogen deficiency on sexual response

- Vaginal blood flow decreased
- Vaginal secretions decreased
- pH increased
- Blood flow to clitoris and labia diminished
- Sensory neurological impairment

Sex in pregnancy

- The physiology remains essentially the same
- Erogenous zones may alter
- Preferred stimulation may alter
- Different positions may be needed for comfortable intercourse

---

1 Johnson AM, Wadsworth J, Wellings K, Field F. *Sexual attitudes and lifestyles.* Oxford: Blackwell Scientific, 1994.
2 Grafenburg E. The role of the urethra in female orgasm. *Int J Sexology* 1950;3:145-8.
3 Masters WH, Johnson VE. *Human sexual response.* Boston, MA: Little, Brown, 1966.

The figures of endocrine regulation of sexual development and internal changes during female sexual response are adapted from Masters WH, Johnson VE, Kolodny RC. *Human sexuality.* 5th ed. New York: Harper Collins, 1995. The female sexual response cycle is adapted from Masters WH, Johnson VE. *Human sexual response.* Boston MA: Little, Brown, 1966. The effect of serum oestradiol on sexual problems is adapted from Sarrel P. Sexuality and menopause. *J Obstet Gynaecol* 1990;75: 265-355. All figures are used with the publishers' permission. The cartoon "No, Son ..." is by Neville Spearman, 1966.

4 Taking a sexual history

John Tomlinson

Many doctors are concerned about their ability to take an appropriate history from a patient with a sexual problem. The main difference from an ordinary medical history is that the patient (and often the doctor) is commonly embarrassed and uncomfortable. Patients may feel ashamed or even humiliated at having to ask for help with a sexual problem that they think is private and that they should be able to cope with themselves. This is particularly so with men, especially young men, who have to admit to erectile dysfunction and therefore, as they see it, the loss of their masculinity. Some hospital doctors get over this initial difficulty by giving patients a preconsultation questionnaire. Many patients like this, but a substantial number dislike its anonymity and apparent coldness.

As with other history taking, the doctor must consider how to put the patient at ease, find out what the real problem is, discover the patient's background and clinical history, and then work out a plan of management with the patient. The doctor should try to avoid showing embarrassment, especially if the patient wants to talk about things that are outside the doctor's experience, as this can cause the patient to clam up.

Above all, there must be sufficient time allowed, and 45–60 minutes is an ideal that is unfortunately not often possible to achieve, although in general practice the patient can be asked to come back for a longer appointment at another time.

Making patients feel comfortable

If the doctor's attitude is matter of fact, then the patient will relax and become matter of fact, too. It must be emphasised that, whatever the patient may admit to, the doctor must be non-judgmental.

A patient's approach to the problem is often tentative and hidden by euphemism, with statements like "I think I need a check up" or "By the way, I have a [discharge, itch, soreness] down below." These comments may well be slipped into a consultation about some other problem, and the doctor has to decide whether to compromise and try to investigate the matter immediately or persuade the patient to come back for a longer consultation.

Various interview techniques can be used to help patients relax more quickly; most are used by many doctors intuitively. These include the manner of greeting a patient, seeing that the patient is seated comfortably, and ensuring privacy and freedom from interuption (especially in a hospital clinic). If the seat is placed at the side of the desk, there is a greater opportunity to observe the patient's body language, as well as this being a more friendly arrangement.

Useful observations on patients' body language include
- their use of their hands and arms—such as uneasily twiddling with a ring, defensively crossing arms, or protectively holding a bag or briefcase on a lap
- a pectoral flush, which creeps over the upper chest and neck (in some younger men as well as women) and which indicates unease despite outward appearance of calm
- the body's position in the chair—the depressed slump, tautly sitting bolt upright, or the relaxed sprawl
- noting postural echo, when doctor and patient sit in mirror images of each other's position—adopted when there is harmony and empathy between the speakers

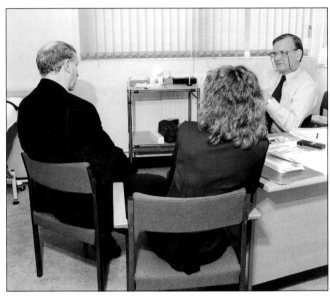

Placing seats at the side of the desk is a more friendly arrangement for an interview and makes it easier to observe a couple's body language to each other, which gives clues to their relationship. (Reproduced with subjects' permission)

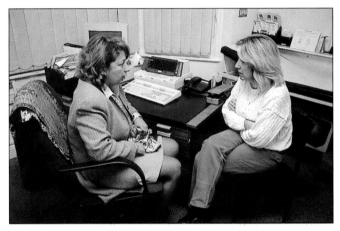

Patients' body language, such as defensively crossing arms, can reveal their state of mind

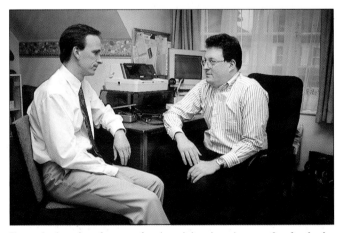

Postural echo, when doctor and patient sit in mirror images of each other's position, indicates empathy between the speakers

Finding out the problem

When people talk about embarrassing subjects, they are often vague and circumlocutory, and what they are trying to say must be clarified. Words such as "impotence," for example, can mean different things to different men (and their partners), including failure to get an erection, failure to maintain an erection, and premature ejaculation, and, equally, a phrase such as "I'm sore down below" can mean anything from pruritus ani to some anatomical problem such as a prolapse or genital warts.

Careful and tactful elucidation is needed, and vagueness must be clarified. The questioner has to be particularly sharp in picking up what the patient is trying to say and be relaxed and unfazed by the subject matter, but this can be overdone.

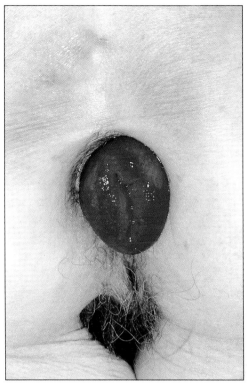

Phrases such as "I'm sore down below" can mean anything from minor irritation to an anatomical problem such as rectal prolapse

> A patient went back to a general practitioner's receptionist to make a new appointment and said, "I don't want to see him again. I only went in with a cold and he asked me all about my sex life."

Very early in the discussion, the patient must be assured of complete confidentiality, particularly with practice and hospital clinic staff, and especially if personal secrets are disclosed, such as extra-marital affairs.

Factors to be noted during the interview include
- The patient's marital state
- How many previous sexual partners there have been and which sex
- Who the current partner is and for how long
- How many children the patient has
- Which of them lives with the patient
- Whether there is obvious stress in the family
- Whether there are financial worries.

Choice of terminology

One difficulty that bothers many doctors is whether to bring vernacular terms into the discussion because of their emotional charge, and some veer to using only medical terms. Patients too, because of embarrassment about using colloquialisms and fear of causing offence, may try to express their problem in medical terms but may well get the meaning wrong. Both can cause problems in getting an accurate history, but doctors must use very careful judgment in deciding if it would be more appropriate to use the language of the streets.

Although there are frank articles in many magazines and newspapers, many patients, especially younger women, still will not know the meaning of "orgasm" but will understand "come." Fellatio and cunnilingus are not words in general use, and use of the street versions would assume a very relaxed and empathic discussion, but "oral sex" is acceptable to men and women of all ages as an alternative. Usually, the line is very fine and is often related to age and gender.

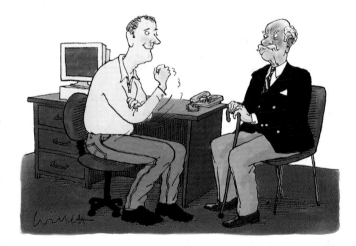

Doctors must use very careful judgment in deciding if it would be appropriate to use colloquialisms when discussing a sexual problem

Open questions

The way open and closed questions are used in history taking is crucial. A closed question expects a specific reply, such as "Yes" or "No," and is characteristic of the medical model of history taking, such as: "Have you had this problem before? Does it hurt when you pass water? Did you practise safe sex?"

Starting with an open question—"How can I help you?"—and continuing with open questions—"What's the problem?" or "What do you think caused the difficulty?"—gives patients an opportunity to expand and to say what is really bothering them. Many younger doctors are worried that a garrulous person might get out of hand, but remaining in control is a skill a good interviewer learns quickly. Judgmental questions—"Don't you think you're past that sort of thing now?"—should be avoided.

> A 16 year old boy was struggling to find medical words to explain his anxieties about masturbation and ejaculation. When the doctor tried to help him out by using colloquial terms the boy looked startled and then grinned and said, "I didn't know doctors knew those words." The rest of the consultation was much more relaxed and informative

Silence

Silence is a powerful tool in taking a good history, and the best interviewers—whether on the radio, on television, or in the consulting room—have realised this. However, many doctors find it extremely difficult not to end a silence, speaking prematurely because they are embarrassed by the quiet or feel that it is rude not to say anything, whereas the patient is often using the time to order his or her thoughts. Valuable details may be lost if those thoughts are cut across by an inappropriate statement from the doctor. The rule is, have patience.

Repetition

Repetition of the last word or phrase, especially if it is one which is emotionally loaded, is a powerful technique to get a patient to elaborate on what he or she is trying to say. Everyone uses this technique, often without thinking, but when it is used deliberately without overtones—although it may seem artificial and forced—it can elicit much information.

Content of a sexual history

Although a joint interview is always much more valuable, patients often prefer to discuss things alone in the first instance. A warm invitation for the partner, coupled with the observation that a sexual problem is not the patient's problem alone, can put the patient's anxieties into perspective.

To be complete, the history must include several factors.

Social history

A detailed social history helps to put the patient into context. The patient's problem can be the first item to be discussed, but taking a social and medical history before exploring the problem allows the patient time to relax while talking about familiar things such as children, home, and job and enables the doctor to put the problems into perspective. Even if the doctor is the patient's general practitioner and knows him or her well, a review of the social history will give a valuable updating and incidental information that is often highly relevant.

Medical history

It used to be thought that all sexual problems, especially erectile dysfunction, were psychogenic in origin. General opinion has shifted to accepting that a large proportion can have a physical basis, though, not surprisingly, often with a psychogenic overlay. It is therefore important to take a detailed medical history, particularly bearing in mind those illnesses that may affect sexual performance.

Diabetes can eventually cause impotence in up to half of affected men.

Depression and psychotic illnesses cause loss of sexual desire (but not necessarily loss of function) in a high proportion of both men and women, but careful questioning is needed to elicit them. Altered sleep pattern is a valuable indicator of depression.

Heart disease, especially when combined with hyperlipidaemia and arteriopathy, accounts for erectile dysfunction in many men.

Other hormone deficiencies, especially thyroid and testosterone, reduce sexual desire and performance in both sexes.

Operations and trauma, especially gynaecological and prostate, can cause problems. Damage to the pelvis or spine is another obvious cause.

Example of using repetition to elicit information

"Doctor, I think I need a check up"
"Yes, of course. It's quite a time since the last one. Let me start with your blood pressure. . . ."

Compare this with
"Doctor, I think I need a check up"
"Check up?"
"Yes, I'm not performing as well as I used to"
"Performing?"
"Yes, well, you know, I think I'm impotent. My wife is very good about it and doesn't complain, but I feel so guilty and ashamed"
"Ashamed?"
"I feel terrible. I don't feel a man any more, especially as we used to have such a good sex life . . . ."

Questions to be asked in sexual history

- The problem as the patient sees it
- How long has the problem been present?
- Is the problem related to the time, place, or partner?
- Is there a loss of sex drive or dislike of sexual contact?
- Are there problems in the relationship?
- What are the stress factors as seen by the patient and by the partner?
- Is there other anxiety, guilt, or anger not expressed?
- Are there physical problems such as pain felt by either partner?

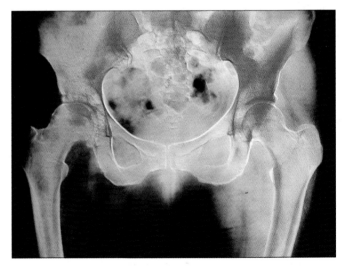

Painful osteoarthritis of the hips or knees limiting movement can be very inhibiting for sexual activity

Prolactinoma may, rarely, present as a loss of sexual desire and headaches in a younger man.

Pain—of arthritis, vaginal atrophy in the older woman, or a phimosis—can be very offputting to one or other partner.

Patient's (and partner's) view of the problem

Marital dysfunction or just plain sexual boredom after many years of being together can be a major cause of impotence. It is useful to try to assess a couple's relationship just by looking at their body language to each other.

In men with erectile dysfunction it is helpful to know the patient's, and especially his partner's, views of the causes as this often reveals their anxieties about other problems, including malignancy. It is also useful to know the speed of onset: organic causes such as diabetes tend to develop slowly whereas psychogenic ones appear more rapidly, but this guide is not infallible. A psychogenic content to the problem is indicated if the man gets erections during the night or on early waking or if he can masturbate successfully—although many are reluctant to admit this in front of their partner. (Erectile dysfunction is covered in a later article in this series.)

Strict upbringing and religious beliefs, especially if there is disparity between the partners as in mixed marriages, can often have a devastating effect on a sexual relationship. Other questions to consider include whether unemployment or the threat of it is causing anxiety, or whether retirement is causing a loss of self esteem in either the patient or partner, with concomitant effects on sexual performance. Has the menopause or a hysterectomy changed the way a woman perceives herself? Does she feel less feminine or attractive to her partner, or has her sex drive increased with freedom from child rearing, causing disparity between the couple's sexual desires and needs?

These aspects may need very tactful questioning to elicit and require sensitivity on the part of the doctor.

Medical and recreational drugs

Many drugs, especially hypotensives, and the quantity and frequency of alcohol and nicotine intake, can have a profound effect on sexual performance, as can many "cold cures" and over the counter hypnotics that contain anticholinergics such as diphenhydramine. Equally, the lack of hormone replacement therapy can cause a major problem in a menopausal woman's sexual relationship, with vaginal atrophy and dryness leading to pain during sexual intercourse. This may not be volunteered by, or even be apparent to, her partner and is a good reason to try to listen to the couple together.

Cannabis can cause an initial euphoria, improving sexual confidence, but, like alcohol, it can greatly diminish ability. Other drugs, including the so called hard drugs, have a deleterious long term effect.

Agreeing a management plan

The final part of history taking is for the doctor to decide what is to be done next. A management plan should then be discussed and agreed with the patient. At this point they should decide whether the patient's partner should be invited for a joint meeting if he or she has not been present. In this way, the patient will feel that a partnership exists with the doctor, and treatment is much more likely to succeed.

The pictures of defensive body posture and postural echo are reproduced with permission of Mike Wyndham. The picture of rectal prolapse, by Dr P Marazzi, and the X ray of an arthritic hip joint, by CRNI, are reproduced with permission of Science Photo Library.

Commonly prescribed drugs associated with sexual dysfunction (list not fully comprehensive)

Drug	Erectile dysfunction	Altered drive	Ejaculatory disorder	Orgasmic disorder	Priapism
Anticonvulsants					
Carbamazepine	✓				
Phenytoin	✓	✓			
Primidone	✓	✓			
Antidepressants					
Tricyclics					
Amitriptyline	✓	✓	✓		
Amoxapine	✓	✓	✓		
Clomipramine	✓	✓	✓	✓	
Imipramine	✓	✓	✓	✓	
Maprotiline	✓	✓			
Nortriptyline	✓	✓			
Protriptyline	✓	✓	✓		
Monoamine oxidase inhibitors					
Phenelzine	✓	✓	✓	✓	
Selective serotonin reuptake inhibitors					
Fluoxetine	✓	✓			
Fluvoxamine	✓	✓			
Paroxetine	✓	✓			
Sertraline	✓	✓			
Antipsychotics					
Chlorpromazine	✓	✓	✓		✓
Fluphenazine	✓	✓	✓		
Haloperidol	✓		✓		
Thioridazine	✓		✓	✓	✓
Benzodiazepines	✓	✓	✓	✓	
Antihypertensives					
Atenolol	✓				
Clonidine	✓		✓	✓	
Guanethidine	✓	✓	✓		
Hydralazine	✓				✓
Labetalol	✓	✓	✓		✓
Methyldopa	✓	✓	✓	✓	
Metoprolol	✓	✓			
Pindolol	✓				
Prazosin	✓				
Propranolol	✓	✓	✓	✓	
Reserpine	✓	✓	✓		
Timolol	✓	✓			
Verapamil	✓				
Diuretics					
Amiloride	✓	✓			
Chlorthalidone	✓	✓			
Indapamide	✓	✓			
Spironolactone	✓	✓			
Thiazides	✓				
Antiemetics					
Metoclopramide	✓	✓			
Non-steroidal anti-inflammatory drugs					
Naproxen	✓		✓		
Anticholinergics					
Atropine	✓				
Diphenhydramine	✓	✓			
Hydroxyzine	✓	✓			
Propantheline	✓				
Scopolamine	✓				
Antispasmodics					
Baclofen	✓		✓		
Hypnotics					
Barbiturates	✓	✓	✓		

Further reading

Morris D. *Man watching*. London: Triad Granada, 1980

Bancroft J. *Human sexuality and its problems*. 2nd ed. Edinburgh: Churchill Livingstone, 1989

Gregoire A, Prior J. *Impotence, an integrated approach to clinical practice*. Edinburgh: Churchill Livingstone, 1993

5 Examination of patients with sexual problems

John Dean

Examining a patient or couple with sexual problems involves standard procedures. However, it can sometimes be fraught with difficulties, often related to psychological and social factors not generally experienced in other situations.

Patients may anticipate the examination with dread and profound embarrassment or, conversely, may see it as a potential source of reassurance and relief. Doctors must be aware of the many popular myths about sex and that their patients may often hold quite idiosyncratic beliefs and fears, which will also need to be addressed.

It is important to explain at the outset how the examination, essential in all patients with a suspected physical problem, might help them and to tell them precisely what it entails. An unusual history, odd behaviour by either partner during assessment, inconsistent findings on examination, or unexplained bruising or trauma may alert you to an abusive relationship. Any suspicions should not be ignored, but great care and sensitivity are needed to address this issue.

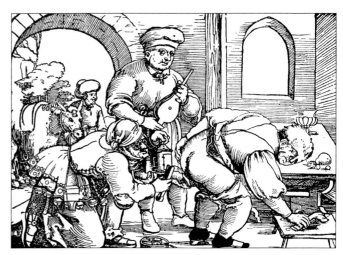

It is important to explain at the outset precisely what an examination entails. (Mercury treatment for venereal disease, circa 1500)

Patient preferences in examination

Many patients will find examination of the genitalia deeply embarrassing. Success will depend on the cooperation and confidence of your patient, and it is best to defer examination if the patient is uncomfortable and unable to relax.

It is good practice to offer to have a chaperone present for both male and female patients if they wish. A substantial minority of patients, both men and women, prefer to be examined by a doctor of their own sex. Remember that patients have made complaints of indecent assault even when their examining doctor was of the same sex.

Cultural differences must also be considered. Many Muslim, Hindu, and Sikh women practise a strict sexual morality. Girls are brought up to be shy and modest, and submitting to a vaginal examination may be regarded with abhorrence, even as a matter of life and death. Remember that our own sexual mores are not universally accepted. It is both wise and a kindness to explore these issues with the patient before proceeding with an examination.

General examination

It is important to make a holistic assessment, not neglecting evidence of concomitant disease that may be a contributory factor to the sexual problem. Cardiovascular, respiratory, or neurological disease may, directly or indirectly, cause sexual problems. Musculoskeletal disorders may lead to sexual problems through chronic pain or immobility. Observe patients' general mobility, spinal mobility, and movement of the hips and knees. A patient's affect may suggest depression, anxiety, or other mental health problems.

The examination of both men and women should include dipstick analysis of the urine for the presence of glucose. Diabetes is a common cause of erectile dysfunction in men and may also cause autonomic neuropathy affecting sexual response. A measurement of fasting blood sugar concentration would be a more reliable option for detecting diabetes if blood has to be taken for other reasons.

Requirements for examination

- Privacy, warmth, and an unhurried approach are essential
- A third of women and a fifth of men prefer to be examined by a doctor of their own sex
- Carefully consider cultural mores
- It is prudent to offer patients a chaperone, both for reassurance and for medicolegal reasons
- Assess patients holistically, excluding other diseases that may have a bearing on their sexual problem such as diabetes, hypertension, and depression

---

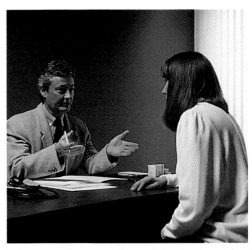

Before examining patients from ethnic minorities, cultural differences in sexual mores should be considered

---

General examination

- Look for evidence of endocrine disease
- Measure blood pressure and perform urine analysis to exclude diabetes
- Check the cardiovascular and central nervous systems
- Examine the abdomen
- Check the external genitalia and, in men, the anus and prostate

---

Examination of male patients

General

Appearance—Observation of general appearance is important and may reveal signs of androgen deficiency or other endocrine abnormalities. The distribution of facial and body hair and the presence of gynaecomastia should be noted. Check blood pressure and radial pulse and palpate the peripheral pulses in men with erectile dysfunction. Evidence of arterial disease, such as the absence of the foot pulses, suggests that an erection problem might be due to arterial insufficiency.

Nervous system—Assess the lumbosacral nervous system if there are indications to do so. There is a dual innervation of the male reproductive system—from the sacral roots (S2-4) through the pudendal and pelvic nerves with predominantly somatic and parasympathetic fibres, and from the thoraco-lumbar roots (T11-L2) through the hypogastric, sympathetic, and pelvic nerves. Tactile (dorsal column) and pinprick (spinothalamic tract) sensation in the perineal and lower limb dermatomes should be assessed. The condition of the perineal reflexes may provide evidence of spinal cord dysfunction.

Abdomen—Check for abdominal surgery or intra-abdominal pathology such as a palpable bladder or kidneys. Hernias may also cause pain and sexual problems.

Testing of reflexes

Perianal reflexes—The muscular contractions provoked in these reflexes can usually be seen or palpated

Bulbocavernosus reflex (S2 and S3)—Firmly squeezing the glans penis provokes a contraction of the bulbocavernosus muscle located between the scrotum and anal sphincter

Bulbo-anal reflex (S3 and S4)—Firmly squeezing the glans penis provokes a contraction of the anal sphincter

Anal reflex (S4 and S5)—Stroking or scratching the skin adjacent to the anus provokes a contraction of the anal sphincter   •

Genital

The appearance of the external genitalia and any apparent developmental anomalies should be noted.

Penis—The size of the flaccid penis is variable, but is usually 5-10 cm in length. It may seem smaller in obese men, being buried in the pubic fat. The presence of any firm plaques of Peyronie's disease should be assessed. The foreskin, if present, should be retracted, and any pain, restriction, or scarring noted. The position of the urethral orifice should be confirmed, and the presence of genital warts or other infective problems noted.

Testes—The testes should feel smooth and symmetrical. The epididymes can be palpated and, again, should be symmetrical and uniform. The vasa should be palpable as firm whipcords, without swellings. A varicocele can sometimes be felt as a swelling above the testicle, more commonly on the left side and is often seen better in the standing position. They are often cited as a cause of fertility problems or pain, but the evidence is inconclusive.

Prostate gland—A rectal examination should be performed (and any perianal problems noted) to assess the size and shape of the prostate. The size of the gland can vary, but it should be firm, smooth, and symmetrical with a uniform consistency (the same firmness as the thenar eminence when the tips of the thumb and forefinger are pressed together), and the median groove should be palpable. It should not be tender to gentle pressure. If it feels hard, irregular, or asymmetrical this suggests prostatic malignancy. Tenderness often indicates prostatitis, which can be a cause of perineal pain or pain on ejaculation. In either case, further investigation is warranted, and referral to a urological or genitourinary medicine specialist should be considered.

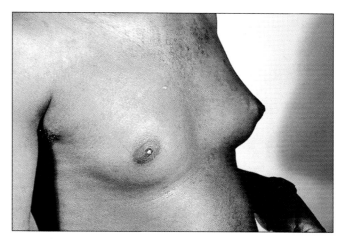

Presence of gynaecomastia should be noted. This usually settles spontaneously but, rarely, may be severe enough to warrant breast reduction

Investigations for male sexual dysfunction

In erectile dysfunction
- Urine analysis for glucose or a blood sugar test to exclude diabetes

In loss of sex drive
- Testosterone (9 am sample)
- Sex hormone binding globulin (SHGP)
- Free androgens (calculated from the above)
- Luteinising hormone (LH)
- Prolactin
- Luteinising hormone and testosterone have a negative feedback relation similar to that of thyroid stimulating hormone and thyroxine. This can be useful in distinguishing hypogonadism and pituitary disorders as causes of testosterone deficiency
- Prostate specific antigen and other investigations are necessary only when coexisting disease is suspected

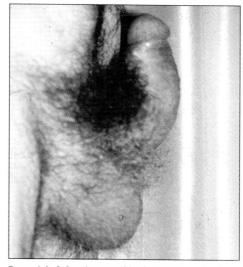

Peyronie's deformity caused by the presence of a dorsal plaque in the penis

Rectal examination

- Look for anal warts, haemorrhoids, sinus, or fissure

The prostate
- Should be smooth and symmetrical with the firmness of a tensed thenar eminence
- May be tender but should not be painful
- Hardness, irregularity, or asymmetry suggests malignancy and needs urgent referral

Examination of female patients

General

As in the male patient, observation of general appearance is important. Assess the development of secondary sex characteristics and exclude hirsutism and other signs of virilisation. Check the blood pressure, radial pulse, and urine. Examine the abdomen and the reflexes including a check of the anal reflex if a neurological problem is suspected.

Genital

Inspect the external genitalia for any apparent developmental anomalies. Note the condition of the labia minora, clitoris, urethral orifice, vagina, and anus and whether there is evidence of warts or other infections. Is the vulval skin healthy or is there evidence of atrophy and oestrogen deficiency? Are hymenal remnants or adhesions present? Note evidence of previous childbirth and scarring from perinatal tears or an episiotomy.

Urinary incontinence—If urinary incontinence related to sexual activity is a problem, it is important to examine the patient with a full bladder. Both stress incontinence and detrusor instability may be the culprit, the latter sometimes being associated with voiding at orgasm. With the patient in the left lateral position, ask her to cough vigorously while you observe the urethral orifice: a jet of urine suggests stress incontinence. If incontinence is a substantial problem referral for urodynamic assessment by a urologist or gynaecologist is prudent.

Speculum examination should be performed, and any pain or vaginal discharge during the procedure should be noted. The appearance of the vagina and cervix should be assessed, and, if appropriate, bacterial and chlamydial swabs may be taken from the vagina and endocervical canal. Excluding chlamydiosis is especially important in women with dyspareunia.

Gentle digital examination of the vagina helps in identifying tenderness and muscle spasm. If tolerated, a bimanual examination should be performed to assess the condition of the cervix, uterus, and adnexa. Particularly note any tenderness, thickening, or swellings. Their presence will often require referral for further assessment by a gynaecologist. The position of the uterus, either anteverted or retroverted, can be noted, but this is rarely of relevance as a cause of sexual problems. Beware of commenting on the position of the uterus to your patient unless you are prepared to address the matter fully.

Rectal examination in a woman is rarely necessary unless an anal or rectal problem is suspected. However, do look at the perianal skin for evidence of scarring, warts, or infection.

Conclusion

When the examination of the patient has been concluded, it is important to give him or her as clear an explanation of the findings as is possible. The findings are often entirely normal, and this reassurance can be very important as a first step in a patient's recovery of his or her sexual wellbeing.

The picture of treating venereal disease is reproduced with permission of Mary Evans Picture Library. The picture of an interview with a patient is reproduced with permission of the Science Photo Library. The picture of gynaecomastia is reproduced with permission of the National Medical Slide Bank. The pictures of speculum, by Simon Fraser, and genital wart are reproduced with permission of Science Photo Library.

Examining a female patient

Examination is necessary only when a physical problem is suspected and may not always be appropriate
- Note the general appearance
- Check secondary sexual characteristics as well as pulse, blood pressure, and urine
- Examine cardiovascular system, central nervous system, abdomen, and external genitalia
- To assess stress incontinence, examine patient with a full bladder and ask her to cough
- Digital and speculum examination of the vagina should be carefully made
- Rectal examination is rarely necessary

Investigations for female sexual dysfunction

Endocrine investigation has limited role but is necessary in women with menstrual irregularity or other symptoms of oestrogen deficiency
- Follicular stimulating hormone and luteinising hormone
- Oestradiol
- Prolactin to exclude a pituitary prolactinoma
- Thyroxine—as in men, hyperthyroidism and hypothyroidism can cause dysfunction in sexual drive and arousal
- Other investigations are necessary only when coexisting disease is suspected

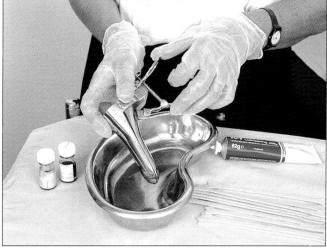

Duck bill speculum used to hold open the vagina during examination and for swabs to be taken

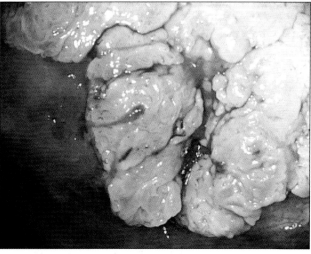

Colposcopy of a genital wart in the cervix

6   Female sexual problems I: Loss of desire—what about the fun?

Josie Butcher

Loss of desire for sexual activity is the commonest presenting female sexual dysfunction and often the hardest to treat. Whether this loss of sexual desire should be seen as abnormal or simply as a variation of normal has long been debated. Much literature is available on female loss of desire, considering sexuality for women from various angles. The American Psychiatric Association's *Diagnostic and Statistical Manual of Mental Disorders* (DSM-IV), which gives our working classification of psychosexual dysfunction, would classify it as hypoactive sexual desire disorder and sexual aversion disorder.

Masters and Johnson's original "human sexual response curve" helps us to understand loss of desire in the context of the normal sexual response. This diagrammatic representation describes increasing sexual pleasure against time—desire for sexual activity followed by arousal, orgasm, and finally resolution. It is important to remember, however, that the physiologies of desire, arousal, and orgasm are separate entities and therefore are not dependent on each other. Women with loss of desire (hypoactive sexual desire disorder) can have good sexual functioning. In essence, they will not initiate sexual contact.

Is desire a thought or a feeling? The answer is not clear, and, certainly early in loving relationships, physical arousal closely follows any sexual thought. Initially, we have a sexual thought, which then facilitates the arousal mechanism through neurological pathways. The thought could be anticipation of the evening ahead or a memory of a previous sexual encounter. Women who do not desire sexual activity can operate quite well sexually once engaged in the sexual encounter. Touch around the clitoris and genital area facilitates neurological pathways, producing good arousal, good lubrication, and on to orgasm.

Causes of loss of desire

Much research into sexual desire is being undertaken, but it is still poorly understood. We know that certain medical conditions affect it. For example depressive illness often dramatically reduces it, as do stress and fatigue.

Organic causes

Testosterone has a part to play in women's sexual desire, although much smaller amounts are required than in men. In women testosterone production is split evenly between the ovaries and the adrenal gland. Androgen deficiency syndrome should be considered after both hysterectomy and bilateral salpingo-oophorectomy, and chemotherapy for cancer, when treatment with testosterone can improve loss of desire. Conditions and drugs that cause hyperprolactinaemia have a direct effect on reducing sexual drive.

The effect of changing hormone patterns at different life stages is poorly understood, but it is well known that loss of desire is more common with premenstrual tension, postnatally, and around the menopause. Many drugs can also cause loss of desire, and it can be secondary to poor sexual arousal and lack of orgasm.

Any health problem that might affect sexual anatomy, the vascular system, the neurological system, and the endocrine system must be considered. Indirect causes are conditions

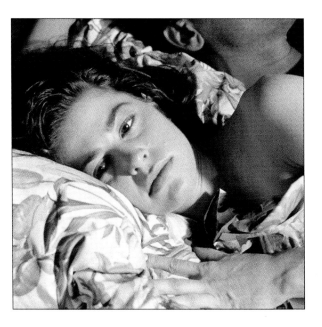

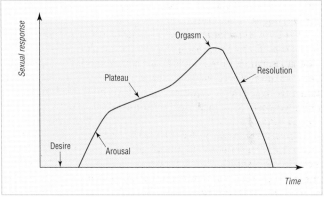

The normal female sexual response. (Adapted from Masters WH, Johnson VE. *Human sexual response*. Boston, MA: Little, Brown, 1966)

Possible causes of hyperprolactinaemia

- Pituitary tumours
- Hypothyroidism
- Cirrhosis
- Stress

- Hypothalamic diseases
- Hepatic disease
- Breast surgery
- Drug treatments

Drugs that can affect women's sexual function

- Antiandrogens
  Cyproterone
  Gonadotrophin releasing hormone
  analogues
- Antioestrogens and other hormones
  Tamoxifen
  Contraceptive drugs

- Cytotoxic drugs
- Psychoactive drugs
  Sedatives
  Narcotics
  Antidepressants
  Neuroleptics
  Stimulants

---

that can cause dyspareunia; that cause chronic pain, fatigue, and malaise; and that interfere with the vascular and neurological pathways.

Psychological causes

It is often difficult to disentangle organic possibilities from psychogenic variables that occur in women at different life stages and the effect that these may have on how women see sexuality fitting into their lives. It is important to consider these points and not to allow ourselves to be dragged into the medical model. We should look at the importance of the different roles that women have in their lives and how they prioritise them.

Many women have several roles—the professional or worker, housewife, mother, daughter, friend, and lover. This last role seems to fade away as the demands of others increase. When a woman meets her first serious partner, she has fewer of these other roles: she may be only a worker and a daughter. In later years, she will have more roles to contend with: she may be a mother and housewife as well. For many women it seems that, as the responsibility of roles increases, the importance of the lover role diminishes.

Looking at these issues can be quite revealing, and an easy way to give structure to this is to undertake a process that we can call the "timetable of life." Both partners in the relationship are asked to fill in a timetable representing a typical week. They are then asked to look at the week in terms of time spent in different categories: family time (that is, with children and partners), work time (both at work and work in the house), extended family time (with parents and relations), social time, personal time, and relationship time (time spent together alone, as a couple). This last category is, of course, the time when sexual activity is more likely to be realised successfully.

A timetable almost always shows the elements missing to be relationship time and personal time. Roles are, of course, not just about the practicalities of who does what but about the responsibilities a woman feels for the roles she takes on.

It is useful to ask a woman her views on her learning about sexuality and the influences that have played a part in the development of her sexuality. Sexual learning and role prioritisation are often intertwined. An example of this is the woman who found that she had lost sexual desire after the birth of her first child. Discussion showed that she had, not unnaturally, made the responsibility of being a mother a high priority, but coupled with this was the clear message that she had received when learning about her sexuality, that "mothers are not sexual beings."

Many misunderstandings and myths can be acquired during learning about sexuality, such as that a man is always ready and able to have sex, that sex is natural and spontaneous, and that sex equals intercourse. Sexual myths are held by women as well as men.

Repeating the "timetable" for different times in a woman's life and comparing it during courtship, when sexual desire was probably good, with the timetable for a time when sexual desire was low is useful and shows how priorities change and how this can influence desire for sexual activity.

Looking at what happens in a sexual situation often gives much information about the defences erected when a patient engages in sexual activity. One can look at what turns a patient on and off, how absorbed she becomes in the sexual experience, and whether loss of desire occurs on every occasion or whether it is situational. Areas such as sexual fantasy, masturbation, genital functioning, and contraception can be discussed and give great insight.

Illnesses that may result in loss of sexual desire

- Gynaecological disorders causing pain on sexual intercourse
- Obstetric disorders causing pain on sexual intercourse
- Urological disorders causing pain on sexual intercourse
- Alcohol and substance misuse
- Stress and chronic anxiety
- Endocrine disorders
- Neurological disorders
- Psychiatric disorders
- Depression
- Fatigue

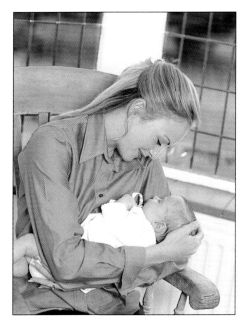

As a woman takes on the roles of mother and housewife, the importance of the lover role may diminish

Possible sources for sexual learning include parental values, religious teaching, cultural mores, and life events

Ten myths about sex

- In general, a man should not be seen to express certain emotions
- In sex, as elsewhere, it is performance that counts
- An erection is essential for a satisfying sexual experience
- All physical contact must lead to sex
- Sex equals intercourse
- Good sex must follow a linear progression of increasing excitement and terminate in orgasm
- Sex should be natural and spontaneous
- On the whole, the man must take charge of and orchestrate sex
- A man wants and is always ready for sex
- We no longer believe the above myths

*Adapted from Zilbergeld B. *Men and sex: a guide to sexual fulfilment.* London: Harper Collins, 1995

Treatment options

An integrated approach to medical and psychological treatments is optimal. Any medical elements of the problem, if present, must be treated to achieve a positive outcome. In secondary loss of desire for sexual activity, a psychogenic aspect often remains after the medical elements have been treated.

Most of the treatment will involve cognitive behavioural approaches and psychodynamic approaches based on the discussions previously described. One of the most difficult areas to approach and deal with is loss of attraction for the partner, which can lead to serious difficulties and consequences.

Working with people as a couple when there is loss of sexual desire allows both partners' understanding of the problem to be examined by means of some of the techniques described above. As partners begin to realise that they can no longer assume that they know how their partner feels, or should feel, the differences in sexuality and sexual needs can be explored. We expect our partners to feel the same way as we feel and to know when we feel sexual. We expect them to be able to provide for our needs sexually without necessarily discussing them. With counselling, the aim is to encourage acceptance of difference, a concept sometimes described as "benign variation."

> Frigidity does not feature in this discussion, nor does it feature in any classification of female sexual dysfunction. The term is more a reflection of women's feelings about themselves or of men's feelings about women. When a woman describes herself as frigid, she is really describing how she feels about herself as a sexual being, and it is often a comparison with her or others' expectations of how she should feel and be. Frigidity is not a medical term, and we should no longer use it.

Further reading

Bancroft J. *Human sexuality and its problems.* 3rd ed. Edinburgh: Churchill Livingstone, 1998
Kaplan HS. *The sexual desire disorders.* New York: Brunner Mazel, 1995
Hawton K. *Sex therapy. A practical guide.* Oxford: Oxford University Press, 1985 (reprinted 1997)
Kitzinger S. *Women's experience of sex.* London: Penguin Books, 1985
Crowe M, Ridley J. *Therapy with couples.* Oxford: Blackwell Science, 1990 (reprinted 1996)
Heiman J, LoPiccolo L, LoPiccolo J. *Becoming orgasmic. A sexual growth programme for women.* New Jersey: Spectrum Books, 1976
Dickson A. *The mirror within.* London: Quartet Books, 1985 (reprinted 1997)
Goodwin AJ, Agronin ME. *A woman's guide to overcome sexual fear and pain.* Oakland, CA: New Harbinger Publications, 1997
Masters WH, Johnson VE. *Human sexual inadequacy.* Boston, MA: Little, Brown, 1970

Diagnostic checklist for women's loss of sexual desire

- Physical illness
  Integrity of anatomy
  Integrity of vascular system
  Integrity of neurological system
  Integrity of endocrine system
- Drugs and treatments
- Psychological characteristics
- Relationship issues
- Life changes
- Sexual history
- Sexual knowledge
- Attraction to partner

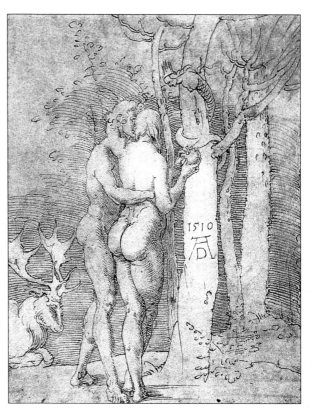

We expect our partners to feel the same way as we feel and to know when we feel sexual. (*Callipygous Eve and Adoring Adam* (1510) by Albrecht Dürer)

The picture of a couple lying in bed is reproduced with permission of Tony Stone Images. The picture of a mother and baby is reproduced with permission of Mother & Baby Picture Library.

7 Female sexual problems II: sexual pain and sexual fears

Josie Butcher

Dyspareunia and vaginismus are two common and extremely frustrating sexual dysfunctions for women. The *Diagnostic and Statistical Manual of Mental Disorders* (DSM-IV) lists them as two separate disorders in the subcategory of sexual dysfunctions.

Dyspareunia

Dyspareunia is recurrent genital pain associated with sexual activity and can be classified as primary, when pain has always occurred during sexual activity, or secondary, when it occurs after a period of pain free lovemaking. The term is usually used to describe pain on penetration, but it can occur during genital stimulation. It is best described according to the site of the pain.

Traditionally, it was thought that superficial dyspareunia (at or around the vaginal entrance) is likely to have a psychogenic origin, whereas deep dyspareunia is likely to have an organic cause. These explanations are no longer considered helpful. It is important to try to identify the history of the pain, its site, sort, severity, onset, duration, and any other associated factors. Look for any physical abnormalities and discuss their effects on the sexual relationship. It must be remembered that physical signs are not always visible, and vulval histology is sometimes required. It is never enough to suggest that dyspareunia is simply psychological, and it should be looked at medically before any psychological components are considered.

Repeated sexual pain can set up a cycle of pain, in which fear of pain leads to avoidance of the sexual activity that produces it, in turn leading to lack of arousal, failure to achieve orgasm, and loss of sexual desire. This can progress to total avoidance of sexual activity and difficulties in the relationship.

Superficial vulval pain

Superficial vulval pain is common and has many causes. Identifying the cause is difficult, however, and patients often see treatments as frustrating and inadequate. There is a great risk of a patient focusing on the discomfort and repeatedly trying to find answers. She may consider herself misunderstood, and her doctor may become frustrated through failure to find a cure. Although patients are anxious and may be introspective about their symptoms, they seem psychologically "healthy."

Vulval pain can be relapsing and remitting. Experiences of burning, itching, and stinging—with patients describing feeling "inflamed"—are common, and any area of the perineum may be affected. Pain may be felt not only on sexual stimulation but can be present all the time and triggered by non-sexual activities such as walking. The main causes are vulvitis, vulvovaginitis, vulvar vestibulitis, vulvodynia, genital herpes, urethritis, and atrophic vulvitis, as well as inadequate lubrication and topical irritants such as spermicides or latex.

Vaginal pain

This is the least common category of dyspareunia, partly because sensory nerve endings are present only in the lower third of the vagina. Pain is mainly experienced at the entrance to the vagina. Common causes are lack of lubrication, vaginal infection, irritants (spermicides and latex), urethral problems, gynaecological and obstetric interventions (episiotomy), radiotherapy (radiation vaginitis), and sexual traumas.

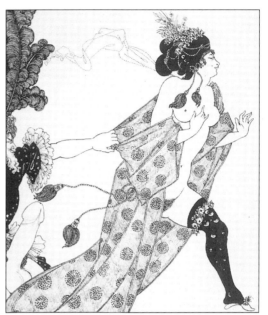

Belief that her vagina is too small may be one of the reasons for a woman's fear of vaginal penetration. (*Cinesias entreating Myrrhina to coition*, 1896, by Aubrey Beardsley)

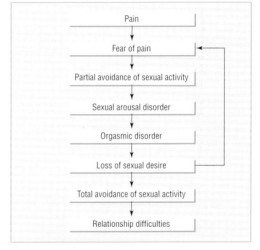

Cycle of sexual pain and avoidance of sexual activity

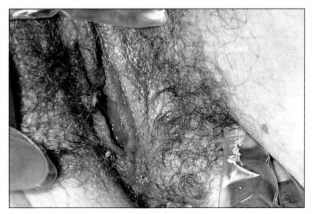

Small sores on vulva caused by herpes simplex II virus. Genital herpes is a major cause of superficial dyspareunia

Deep dyspareunia

Deep dyspareunia, often described as pain resulting from pelvic thrusting during sexual intercourse, is also common and has many causes. Major causes include pelvic inflammatory disease; gynaecological, pelvic, or abdominal surgery; postoperative adhesions; endometriosis; genital or pelvic tumours (including fibroids); irritable bowel syndrome; urinary tract infections; and ovarian cysts. A common cause is positional, with deep thrusting by the woman's partner hitting an ovary (equivalent to hitting or squeezing a man's testicle).

Treatment

When considering treatments for dyspareunia, all physical causes should be treated as far as possible. However, cognitive behavioural programmes can be useful and are similar to the approach used for vaginismus (see below). Many women, once they understand their sexual problem, can adapt and can achieve good quality sexual activity leading to penetration even though they have a painful physical condition. Successful treatment is in large measure due to the patient feeling that she owns her vagina and controls her sexual activity.

Vaginismus

This is a conditioned response that results from associating sexual activity with pain and fear. It is a severe problem for many women, who may experience not only extreme physical pain on attempted penetration but also severe psychological pain. It consists of a phobia of penetration of the vagina and involuntary spasm of the pubococcygeal and associated muscles surrounding the lower third of the vagina.

Primary vaginismus is diagnosed when a women has never experienced vaginal penetration, and secondary vaginismus is diagnosed when a woman has had vaginal penetration without a problem in the past.

The severity of the symptoms can lead to a general sexual inhibition with avoidance of any sexual touching, and in most severe cases to avoidance of any affectionate touching. The spasm can occur not only on attempted penetration but on anticipated penetration or foreplay. At the other end of the spectrum some women are sexually responsive and have good quality sexual experiences, with imaginative "foreplay" continuing to orgasm but avoiding penetration.

Attempted penetration leads to pain, fear, humiliation, and frustration, often resulting in feelings of inadequacy and abandonment. The discomfort from repeated attempts at penetration or speculum examination can produce a tightening of muscles in the pelvis, thighs, abdomen, and legs. As well as unsuccessful intercourse, women will have experienced failed gynaecological examinations, difficulty using tampons, and defaulting from attendance for cytology of cervical smears, all of which are almost impossible.

Causes

The immediate cause of vaginismus, whether primary or secondary, is the involuntary muscle spasm. Why some women develop vaginismus and others do not is uncertain. The initial response may be secondary to any type of vaginal pain, including all causes of dyspareunia. Experience of physical or sexual abuse can induce phobia of vaginal penetration, as can frightening medical procedures experienced during childhood, painful first sexual intercourse, problems with a relationship, and fear of pregnancy.

Masters and Johnson suggested that important factors may include religious orthodoxy, poor sexual education, sexual inhibition, sexual abuse, rape, and anger in relationships.

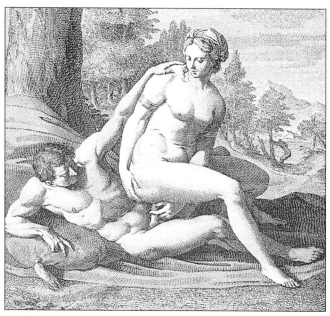

By taking complete control of vaginal penetration, women can learn to overcome their fear of sexual activity. (*Angelique et Medor* from *Aretino or The Loves of the Gods*, circa 1602, by Agostino Carracci)

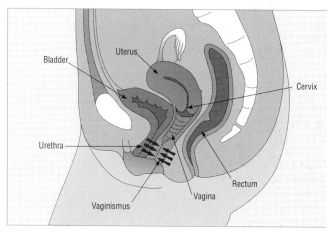

Diagram of vaginismus. (Redrawn from Masters WH, Johnson VE, Kolodny RC. *Human sexuality.* 5th ed. New York: Harper Collins, 1995)

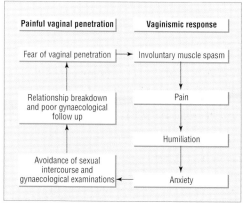

Cycle of vaginismus

Other suggested factors include fear of intimacy, pregnancy, or aggression and belief that one's vagina is too small. There is a suggestion that psychological conflict can be implicated, in which a woman indirectly expresses anger towards her partner by closing off her vagina.

Treatment

Cognitive behavioural treatment programmes for vaginismus comprise a programme of relaxation with specific exercises for relaxing the muscles around the vagina and a systematic desensitisation of the vagina.

The woman learns to control her vaginal muscle spasm while gently introducing trainers of gradually increasing size into the vagina. Trainers can be fingers, tampons, or specifically designed specula such as Simms or Amielle. Throughout, the woman is in total control, and this gives her great confidence. The programme progresses to a point where she is able to share the introduction of the trainers with her partner. This stage is followed by insertion of the penis into the vagina with the woman in control.

The phobic element of the problem also needs to be addressed and is often the most difficult part of the treatment. Although women may dread the prospect of the treatment programme, the success rate is nearly 100% if the woman persists with the programme. The aim of the treatment is to achieve a situation where the woman feels that she owns her own vagina and can share it for sexual activity should she wish.

Anorgasmia (female orgasmic disorder)

The role of orgasm for women is not well defined. For some it is extremely important and sought at every sexual encounter. However, for others it seems less important and sometimes of little relevance; many women can be quite content without it. An important issue is the male partner's understanding of the female orgasm. He often feels that, like him, his partner cannot fully enjoy sexual activity without orgasm, and this can put enormous pressure on the woman to achieve orgasm.

A working definition of anorgasmia would be an involuntary inhibition of the orgasmic reflex. A woman may have a strong sexual desire with good arousal and enjoy the sensation of the penis in the vagina, but she then holds back even though the stimulation should be sufficient for orgasm. These women often have a strong fear of losing control over feelings and behaviour. The fear can be conscious or unconscious, but resolution of the conflict is an important aim of treatment. An example of a situational anorgasmia is a woman who can achieve orgasm by masturbation but not in coupled sexual activity.

Historically, orgasm has been equated with loss of control leading to death and has been described as the "mini-death." Most women coming for help feel that having an orgasm will dramatically change their lives. Education and rational discussion is important in disassociating orgasm from symbolic qualities.

Treatment

Work with both the individual and the couple is aimed at treating the "holding back"—the fear or phobia of orgasm or losing control. Resolution of conflicts (decreasing inhibitions) combined with increasing stimulation is very successful.

A considerable amount of couple work is helpful, during which sexual education, sexual myths, and a greater understanding of a partner's needs can be discussed. The question, "Who is this orgasm for?" can be addressed. The idea of difference can be achieved, and the concept of benign variation of sexual need accepted.

Treating vaginismus

1—Sexual education
2—Control of vaginal muscles
3—Self exploration of sexual anatomy
4—Insertion of a trainer under controlled relaxation
5—Sharing of control with partner
6—Insertion of penis, with the woman in control
7—Transfer control of insertion of penis to partner
8—Exploration of phobia

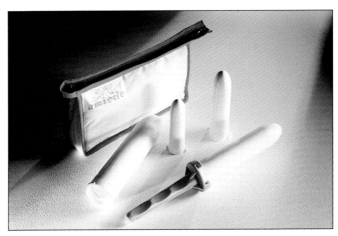

Amielle trainers, which can be used to help overcome fear of vaginal penetration

---

Classification of anorgasmia

Primary—Orgasm has never been achieved
Secondary—Orgasm has been achieved in the past
Absolute—Orgasm impossible in all situations
Situational—Orgasm impossible only in certain situations

Treating anorgasmia

1—Self exploration	2—Sensate focus
3—Masturbation	4—Use of adjuncts (vibrators)
5—Resolution of unconscious fears of orgasm	6—Distraction
7—Exercises to heighten sexual arousal	8—Transfer to heterosexual situation
9—Orgasm on sexual intercourse	

Objectives of treatment

- Heightening sexual arousal so that woman is close to orgasm before penetration
- Enhancing awareness of pleasure and vaginal sensation with tactile stimulation in outer third of the vagina
- Maximising clitoral stimulation with active thrusting by woman, woman in superior position, direct clitoral stimulation, use of a vibrator, and use of external clitoral stimulation by woman

---

The picture of genital herpes, by Dr P Marazzi, is reproduced with permission of Science Photo Library.

8 A woman's sexual life after an operation

Asun de Marquiegui, Margot Huish

Disfiguring and mutilating operations, especially of the face, breasts, genitals, and reproductive organs, often have a deleterious effect on a woman's self image and sexuality. Sociopsychological aspects of body image form a complex pattern of self knowledge and how one is perceived by others. The invasion of surgery invariably causes temporary or permanent changes, which may not be anticipated by women or may emerge only on discharge from hospital.

Partners who adapt poorly to the new circumstances may also find it difficult to continue sexual activity, but an existing strong and intimate relationship encourages positive postoperative adjustment.

Dealing with psychological and emotional states such as anxiety, fear, and depression about surgery is crucial to a woman and her partner. Medical teams should encourage women to discuss their worries, especially sexual anxieties, as problems become more entrenched and more difficult to treat over time. Postoperative surveys of women suggest that 28–50% wanted their doctor to address sexual difficulties. Rehabilitation is important in promoting adjustment and acceptance by facilitating the grieving process.

Ileostomy, colostomy, and urostomy

Women who have a stoma as a result of chronic illness such as irritable bowel disorder, ulcerative colitis, and Crohn's disease often experience a better psychological and sexual outcome than do those who undergo emergency surgery for, say, cancer of the colon. Healthy adaptation to a stoma depends on preoperative and postoperative counselling and understanding by stoma nurses. Patients' greatest fears are loss of control, bad odour, noise, leaking or bursting bags, unsightliness, and their partner's feelings towards them.

It can be some time before a couple resumes love making after surgery, particularly if attention is focused on the patient's survival or if there are complications such as ill fitting appliances, parastomal sepsis, and skin excoriation. Dyspareunia can be a major problem, not only because of lack of arousal or secondary vaginismus after surgery but because of the amount of scar tissue within the pelvis.

Hip surgery

Total or partial hip replacement is now a common operation, but when a patient can safely resume sex is often not mentioned. Anatomically, internal rotation is dangerous postoperatively because it can lead to dislocation, but, as intercourse usually requires external rotation of the joint, sex can generally be resumed when the scar is comfortable.

Heart operations and angina

While these are often done as lifesaving operations with very good outcomes, women must be allowed to discuss their fears about when or if it is safe to restart sexual activity. Intercourse can take place when a woman feels like it, provided she can walk up two flights of stairs without difficulty, the equivalent cardiac output of orgasm. Angina may limit her activity, although this is unlikely. After a chest operation, she should take the female superior or another comfortable position until discomfort from the chest scar has eased.

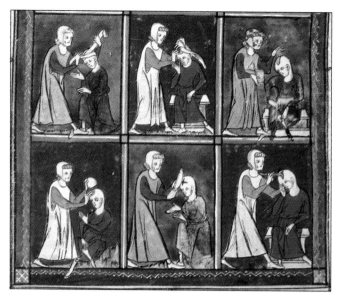

Disfiguring operations, especially of the face and sexual organs, often have a deleterious effect on a woman's self image and sexuality. (Detail from *On Surgery* (14th century manuscript) by Rogier de Salerne)

Factors affecting sexual function after an operation

- Disfigurement or mutilation altering the body image
- Previous psychological and emotional states
- Physical pain and hormonal, vascular, or nervous damage
- Existing problems with intimacy and quality of relationship

---

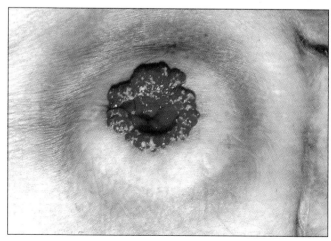

Healthy adaptation to a stoma depends on adequate counselling for both the patient and her partner

Eye operations

Cataract removal places no restrictions on sexual activity, but intercourse should be avoided for two weeks after a retinal detachment, and patients with vitreous haemorrhages need to wait until their laser treatment has finished or, if they do not have diabetes, two weeks after the bleeding has stopped.

Gynaecological operations

Hysterectomy

The uterus, menstruation, and fertility are seen by many women as fundamental to their femininity. After hysterectomy women often have great difficulty becoming sexually aroused, particularly when there are signs of depression before the operation and the woman is aged under 40. However, in some women, for whom other treatments have not worked, hysterectomy can be a relief from heavy bleeding, pain, and tiredness, allowing a freer sexual life.

Intercourse is usually avoided for six weeks, but this is somewhat arbitrary. Gentle penetration is quite possible after four weeks, although many women prefer to wait longer.

Vaginal repairs

These are done mainly for prolapse of the bladder or rectum. Some women complain of postoperative vaginal tightness or dyspareunia because of tender scar tissue. They should be encouraged to restart sexual intercourse when it feels comfortable, using a water based lubricant such as KY jelly or Senselle or an aromatic oil such as peach kernel or sweet almond oil (though oils must not be used with barrier contraceptives made from latex rubber as they will render them ineffective).

Incontinence and colloid injections

Sexual expression can be badly affected by incontinence, with fears about odour, leakage, and wetness. If a woman tenses her pubococcygeal muscles and bladder sphincter in order not to dribble urine, the resulting physiological and psychological tension can lead to vaginismus and possibly dyspareunia and interference with sexual arousal and orgasm.

Minor operations

The diagnosis of an abnormal cervical smear can create great anxiety, especially when it is totally unexpected. It is important to let a woman express her anxiety and fears about cervical cancer and its effect on her sex life before referring her for colposcopy. She will then find it easier to resume her sexual life after treatment.

Female genital mutilation

This operation is illegal in Britain, but the obstetric and sexual sequelae are seen in clinics in areas with large African and Middle Eastern communities. Recent arrivals may need deinfibulation because they are getting married or are pregnant. Young women brought up in Britain may feel mutilated compared with their peers. They need appropriate sexual counselling, and occasionally deinfibulation. Problems with non-consummation of marriage are common, often due to vaginismus. It is important that these women are examined by doctors comfortable with treating psychosexual problems.

Episiotomies, obstetric tears, and trauma

Episiotomies are routinely done to prevent tears in the perineum during labour. It is essential that midwives and

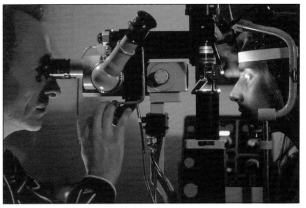

Patients undergoing laser treatment for a detached retina or vitreous haemorrhage should be warned to avoid sexual activity

Example of a case history:

A 49 year old housewife of average intelligence came to a family planning clinic eight weeks after undergoing a hysterectomy because she was worried about not having had a period yet and to find out when she could resume sexual intercourse. She had not felt able to ask at the gynaecology clinic because everyone was so busy

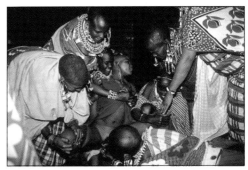

African girl undergoing ritual circumcision (photographed with subjects' permission)

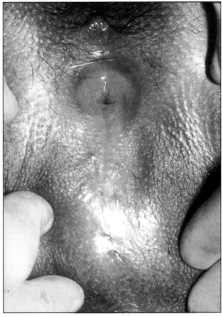

Examination of a woman who had undergone ritual genital mutilation as a child and who now requires deinfibulation to enable her to reproduce

junior doctors are properly trained and take great care in the site and length of incision and its repair to protect the perineum. Poor repairs that lead to painful scars, malposition of the sutures, narrowing of the introitus, or even extrusion of pieces of catgut can severely affect sexual pleasure.

Since low sexual desire, dyspareunia, and secondary vaginismus are common responses after childbirth, women may benefit from postnatal referral to a therapist to discuss sexual dysfunction. Psychological reasons are varied, but tiredness, especially when breast feeding, and fears of a further pregnancy can also have a negative effect on a sexual relationship. A woman's focus on her body as a mother rather than as a lover can also affect sexual function.

Termination of pregnancy

Some women feel relieved after a termination, and it has little impact on their psychological wellbeing, but others may feel a deep sense of loss and grief. This causes anxiety, depression, loss of sexual desire, and difficulties within an existing relationship. When this happens, the reasons why the termination was wanted need to be explored, and all the emotions of that loss need to be counselled. Intercourse can be resumed when the woman has stopped bleeding after the termination if she feels like it.

Sterilisation

Women aged over 30 who have completed their family, and especially those who have had problems with contraception, may find that their sexual activity improves after elimination of the possibility of unwanted pregnancies, and they can resume intercourse as soon as they feel physically comfortable after the operation. On the other hand, women coerced for family or other reasons into unwanted sterilisation may retreat sexually.

Operations for infertility

The pressure to perform to a calendar gives rise to many sexual problems for both men and women. The low success rate of treatments also increases the feelings of failure, loss, grief, frustration, and depression. Couples need counselling to maintain their sexual intimacy while undergoing medical and surgical interventions and beyond.

Operations for cancer

Operations such as hysterectomy, bilateral oophorectomy, and radical vulvectomy can cause major genital mutilation, often producing difficult psychosexual problems. Women have to deal not only with the fear and anxiety of the diagnosis and treatment, but with the constant fear of recurrence. They often do not know what to expect sexually after an operation because of lack of communication with their doctors as well as with their partners.

Partners mainly suffer in silence and find it difficult to make sexual approaches. They fear being seen as selfish or not understanding the physical and emotional pain that the woman is going through if they do, or they may put more pressure on her by assuming that she does want sex. Some partners find that they cannot cope with the physical differences caused by the operation, and this makes restarting a sexual life a big ordeal.

A recent study showed that 75% of women who had undergone radical vulvectomy or radical hysterectomy had sexual difficulties for more than six months postoperatively, and 15% never resumed sexual intercourse. Women who were aged under 50 or not sexually experienced and those not in a relationship at the time of the operation were worst affected. The most common problem was lack of sexual arousal.

A frank preoperative discussion is essential, and the women's partner should be involved from the beginning. If

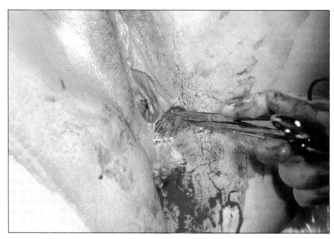

Exploration of a six month old episiotomy scar to remove a painful granuloma, probably the result of stitch that was not removed after the original procedure

---

Possible negative experiences after termination of pregnancy

- Avoidance, denial, feelings of numbness or worthlessness
- Anger, tearfulness, depression
- Dissociation from body, negative thoughts and feelings
- Recurrent intrusive thoughts, flashbacks, dreams and nightmares
- Guilt, shame, detachment, loss of positive feelings
- Suicidal thoughts, feelings of loss of control
- Psychological problems (eating disorders, etc)
- Disinterest in and avoidance of sex, possible vaginismus
- Symptoms can be immediate, delayed, or chronic

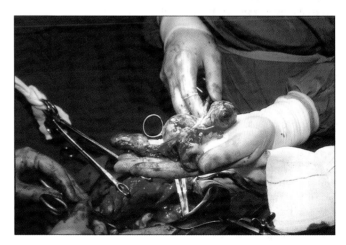

Removal of a woman's uterus and ovaries because of cervical or uterine cancer can lead to psychosexual problems in addition to the fear of the diagnosis and treatment

---

Minimising psychosexual problems after gynaecological operations for cancer

- Try to involve the partner
- Avoid radiotherapy if possible
- Minimise physical mutilation
- Preserve ovarian function
- Reconstruct vagina if possible
- At follow ups check sexual activity
- Refer for sexual counselling

at all possible, radiotherapy should be avoided in order to minimise the physical mutilation and to preserve the ovaries. At every follow up visit all women should be asked how their sexual life is progressing, and sexual counselling should be offered early to minimise long term damage.

Discussion and management

Before an operation takes place it is essential to discuss with the woman, and preferably with her partner, the full implications of the operation on their sexual life. To allow the full expression of their fears, myths, gains, and losses, discussions should be conducted in private in a frank and empathic way. This helps to minimise sexual dysfunction after the operation.

Postoperatively, permission giving and the importance of starting sexual activity early should be emphasised. If a woman has had radiotherapy, oestrogen cream should be used in the vagina. Different positions for intercourse may have to be tried to lessen dyspareunia. Clinical depression should be treated first. When there are intrinsic difficulties with a relationship, the couple should be counselled by an appropriately trained person.

Before surgery, some couples may have chosen not to be sexually active, and this must be taken into account when discussing sexual activity before and after the operation. Good communication skills, especially good listening skills, are essential if a doctor is to show empathy, respect, and non-judgmental attitudes when discussing sexual issues with patients.

Mastectomy, breast enlargement and reduction

The reason for undergoing a mastectomy is all important when considering the effect it can have upon a woman and her sex life. Cancer and fear of it returning, chemotherapy and radiotherapy with their side effects, can all cause a negative body image in addition to depression and a feeling of lowered sexual worth. Arm movement may be restricted and the lopsided feel to the body, even when wearing a prosthesis, can be a constant reminder of the surgery and its cause. The resulting postoperative disfigurement can be far greater than the patient expected, and a thorough explanation before and after surgery by the surgical team, which should include a skilled counsellor, is needed to restore confidence and regain a good enough body image to enter into a relaxed and trusting sexual relationship. Her partner's response and support is all important as a predictor to a healthy sexual outcome. Whether the breasts were of particular importance during lovemaking before surgery can also change the outcome, as scarring and acceptability of shape can be problematic for the woman and her partner.

On the other hand, mastectomy can also be a great relief and a physical and sexual necessity for biological women who are undergoing gender reassignment, and can produce good sexual results because of resultant high self esteem and body image (see also the chapter on sex variations by de Silva).

Enlargements or alternatively reductions can offer relief and freedom from previous anxiety, especially if the feelings about the original size were reinforced by the woman's partner, but there can be anxieties about the outcome in terms of unexpected difference and scarring. However, if the woman is dysmorphophobic and has a fear of being deformed, the results may make little difference to her prior anxieties and depressed state. Loss of the expected post-operative euphoria can further depress her, greatly affecting sexual expression.

Discussing the implications of a gynaecological operation

- Explain possible risks to sexuality
- Allow expression of fears, myths, gains, and losses
- Facilitate communication between partners
- Help to increase intimacy
- Genital sex is not the only form of sex
- Explore other forms of sex and intimacy
- Offer appropriate support

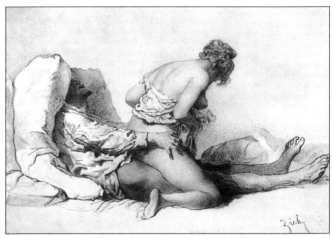

After an operation, different positions for intercourse may have to be tried to lessen dyspareunia. (Man and woman making love, from *Love* (1911) by Mihaly von Zichy)

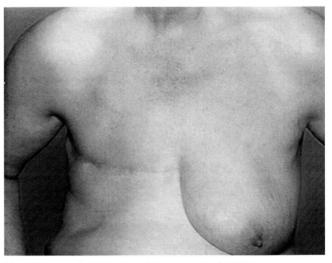

The manuscript by Salerne and the engraving by Zichy were reproduced with permission of the Bridgeman Art Library. The photographs of a stoma, of eye surgery (by Phillip Hayson), of female genital mutilation (by James Stevenson), of granuloma in an episiotomy scar (by PtMarazzi), and of hysterectomy (by Antonia Reeve) were reproduced with permission of Science Photo Library. The photograph of a girl undergoing ritual circumcision was reproduced with permission of Carol Beckwith and Angela Fisher.

Further reading

Crowther ME, Corney RH, Shepherd JH. Psychosexual implications of gynaecological cancer. *BMJ* 1994;308:869-70.

Help with sexual problems

A list of clinics and practitioners is available from the British Association for Sexual and Marital Therapy, PO Box 13686, London SW20 9ZH

9 Male sexual function

Roger S Kirby

Normal sexual function is something most men take for granted. When sexual dysfunction develops, however, stress and anxiety result, which often compound the problem. Relationship difficulties may follow when the partner misinterprets fading erectile prowess as a sign of diminished affection. The quality of life of all those concerned is often adversely affected.[1] In order to understand why sexual function in men is so vulnerable, it is necessary to consider the relevant anatomy and physiology of the normal man.

Anatomy of sexual function

The key structures mediating sexual function in men are the paired corpora cavernosa of the penis (the erectile bodies), which consist of two cylinders with robust fibrous walls (the corpora albuginea). Attached firmly to the ischial tuberosities of the pelvis on each side, the corpora fuse distally in the midline for three quarters of their length.

In the ventral groove formed by both corpora lies the corpus spongiosum, also with erectile capacity. This surrounds the urethra, which runs the length of the penis within this structure. Distally, the corpus spongiosum expands to form the glans penis.

The three erectile bodies are surrounded by Buck's fascia, a robust elastic layer, which is surrounded by the superficial penile, or Colles, fascia. Enclosing all is the penile skin, which is remarkably moveable and expandable to accommodate the necessary expansion during erection. Distally, the skin of the penis is attached to the glans to form the prepuce or foreskin.

The erectile tissue of both the corpora cavernosa and the corpus spongiosum consists of multiple lacunar spaces, interconnected and lined by vascular endothelium. The trabeculae form the walls of these spaces and are composed of a mixture of smooth muscle and a fibroelastic framework of collagen.[2]

Vascular anatomy

Erection is a haemodynamic event. The blood supply to the corpora stems mainly from the internal pudendal arteries as the paired branches of the internal iliac arteries.

The cavernosal artery pierces the tunica, enters each corpus cavernosum at the hilum of the penis, and runs distally near the centre of each erectile body. It gives off numerous terminal branches, the helicine arteries, which are corkscrew shaped and open directly into the lacunar spaces. The walls of these resistance vessels consist of smooth muscle, and they act as sphincter mechanisms. When the penis is flaccid this muscle is contracted, allowing only small amounts of blood into the lacunar spaces. After erotic stimuli, however, the helicine arteries dilate, increasing blood flow and pressure to the lacunar spaces.

Three systems drain venous blood from the penis during detumescence: superficial, intermediate, and deep. The superficial system drains blood from multiple superficial veins of the skin and subcutaneous tissue above Buck's fascia. The intermediate system lies beneath Buck's fascia and consists of the deep dorsal vein and its circumflex branches. The deep drainage system comprises the cavernosal and crural veins. All systems eventually empty into the iliac venous system.

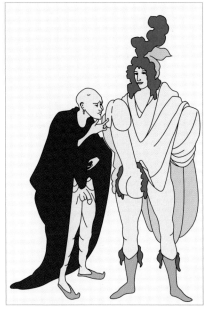

It is necessary to consider the relevant anatomy of the normal man. (*The Examination of the Herald* (1896) by Aubrey Beardsley)

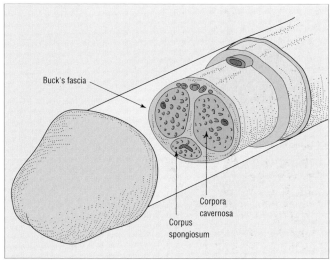

Cross section of the penis showing the corpora cavernosa, corpus spongiosum and Buck's fascia

Buck's fascia

Corpora cavernosa

Corpus spongiosum

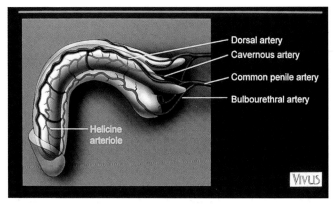

Arterial supply to the penis

Dorsal artery
Cavernous artery
Common penile artery
Bulbourethral artery
Helicine arteriole

VIVUS

Drainage of the corpora cavernosa is by way of venules located at the periphery of the erectile tissue forming a network under the tunica albuginea. These venules coalesce to form the emissary veins, which pierce the tunica and drain mainly by way of the circumflex veins into the deep dorsal vein.

Compression of the subtunical venules by expansion of the trabecular structures against the sturdy tunica albuginea causes a dramatic increase in resistance to blood outflow from the corpora. This is known as the veno-occlusive mechanism and is triggered by relaxation of trabecular smooth muscle. This mechanism allows the maintenance of high intracavernosal pressure with only minor further inflow. The system is so efficient that outflow resistance increases 100-fold compared with that during flaccidity. Once erection has been established only 1–5 ml of blood are required to maintain intracavernosal pressures within the physiological range of 60–100 mm Hg.

Neuroanatomy

Three sets of nerves are involved in normal male sexual function: thoraco-lumbar sympathetic ($T_{11} - L_2$), lumbo-sacral parasympathetic ($S_2 - S_4$), and lumbosacral somatic ($S_2 - S_4$). Somatic sensory fibres travelling via the pudendal nerves convey penile sensation. Cell bodies in the sacral spinal cord situated in Onuf's nucleus relay with parasympathetic connections from the intermediolateral grey matter of the spinal cord. Ascending fibres transmit sensation centrally to diverse areas in the brain which modulate erection.

The "sacral erection centre" consists of preganglionic parasympathetic cell bodies whose fibres extend to the pelvic plexus, where they synapse. Postganglionic parasympathetic fibres pass forward in the cavernous nerves posterolateral to the prostate to innervate the corpora. The cavernous nerves also carry sympathetic postganglionic fibres which supply not only the corpora cavernosa but also the bladder neck, prostate, and seminal vesicles.

Physiology of erection

The penis acts as a capacitor during erection, accumulating blood under pressure within the corpora. The helicine arteries are contracted when the penis is flaccid, creating a pressure gradient between the cavernosal artery and the lacunar spaces.

Dilatation of the cavernosal and helicine arteries is the primary event leading to penile erection.[3] In the normal potent man a twofold dilatation of the cavernosal artery can be detected by colour Doppler ultrasound scanning, as well as a dramatic increase in peak flow velocity to more than 30 cm/sec. The dilated blood vessels allow transmission of systemic pressure to the corpora. Progressively, the penis expands and elongates, and intracavernosal pressure begins to rise.

Relaxation of the trabecular smooth muscle enables the filling and dilatation of the lacunar spaces with expansion of the erectile tissue against the tunica albuginea. Compression of the subtunical venules prevents egress of blood from the corpora, further increasing intracorporeal pressure.

The penis widens and elongates to its maximal capacity, but once the compliance limit for its fibroelastic elements have been reached intracavernosal pressure rises rapidly. Once it rises above diastolic values blood flow occurs only during systole. At maximum rigidity, intracavernosal pressure equilibrates at the cavernosal artery's systolic occlusion pressure less the loss of pressure from venous corporal drainage.

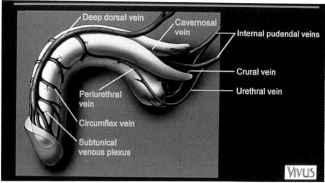

Venous drainage of the penis

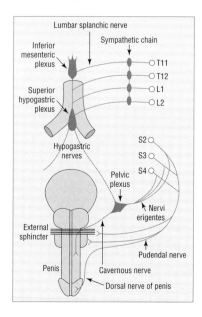

Nerve supply of the penis

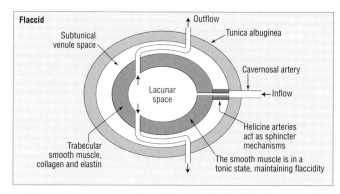

(a) Diagrammatic representation of blood flow in flaccid and erect penis. For the sake of simplicity, all lacunar spaces are treated as one entity.

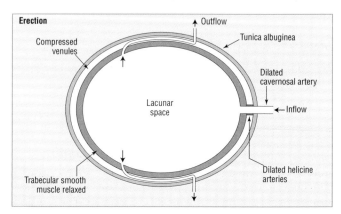

(b) Relaxation of trabecular smooth muscle enables filling and dilation of the lacunar space with expansion of erectile tissue against the tunica albuginea.

Regulation of cavernosal smooth muscle contractility

The smooth muscle of the penis is the key factor in the haemodynamic events that govern erection. About 45% of cavernosal volume is smooth muscle, the non-muscular component being mainly composed of collagen.

The maintenance of flaccidity depends on active contraction of the helicine arteries which in turn depends on the phosphorylation of myosin by adenosine triphosphate (ATP). This permits the formation of attachments between actin and myosin, which permit prolonged maintenance of smooth muscle tone. This state of tone is critically dependent on a high concentration of cytoplasmic free calcium.

Relaxation of the smooth muscle of the helicine arteries and the walls of the intracorporeal trabeculae is accomplished by a lowering of cytoplasmic free calcium. There are several mechanisms by which this can be achieved, but all ultimately depend on the accumulation of one or other of the high energy cyclic nucleotides, cyclic adenosine monophosphate (cAMP) or cyclic guanosine triphosphate (cGTP). Recently, nitric oxide (NO) has been shown to activate guanosine triphosphatase (GTPase), producing cyclic guamosine mono-phosphate (cGMP), which subsequently triggers the lowering of intracellular free calcium. Nitric oxide is produced as a neurotransmitter substance by nitric oxide synthetase in parasympathetic nerve endings and endothelial cells within the corpora.[4] cGMP is broken down by type 5 phosphodiesterase (PDE_5). Sildenafil, a specific inhibitor of PDE_5 therefore potentiates the effect of NO and enhances the erectile response in men suffering from erectile dysfunction when taken orally. Other muscle relaxants such as prostaglandin E_1 and vasoactive intestinal peptide (VIP), given by injection in the treatment of erectile dysfunction also act via mechanisms dependent on cAMP, again by reducing intracellular levels of calcium. Phentolamine, another oral facilitator of erection is an α_1 and α_2 adrenergic angatonist. Vasodilation is caused by the combined α blockade.

Counterbalancing the vasodilatory effects of these and other transmitters are vasoconstrictory influences such as noradrenaline released from sympathetic nerve terminals. These act to increase cytoplasmic free calcium and are important not only for maintaining flaccidity but for inducing detumescence after ejaculation. Since ejaculation itself is sympathetically mediated, resulting in closure of the bladder neck and contraction of the prostate and seminal vesicles, it is easy to see how active contraction of the helicine arteries naturally follows this event; intracorporeal pressure therefore declines, and the veno-occlusive mechanisms reverse. This is the mechanism by which detumescence is achieved.

Conclusions

Normal male sexual function requires penile erection, which is a neurogenic and haemodynamic event. The microanatomy and molecular physiology of this process has recently been clarified. Normal erectile activity depends on intracorporeal smooth muscle function, which is controlled by a balance of vasoconstrictory and vasodilatory neurotransmitter substances modulating cytoplasmic calcium levels in penile smooth muscle.[5] In view of the complexity of these mechanisms it is unsurprising that a wide variety of disorders can result in male erectile dysfunction (ED). These, and the remedies for them, are the subject of other chapters.

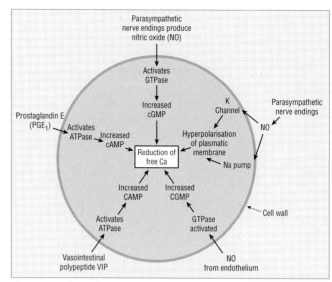

Neurotransmitter substances controlling intracorporeal smooth muscle contractility by modulating cytoplasmic free calcium

---

Mechanisms of lowering the intracellular free calcium

Reduction of intracellular free calcium lowers the state of tone and enables the smooth muscle cell to relax. The main muscle relaxants are nitric oxide (NO), prostaglandin E_1 (PGE_1) and vasointestinal polypeptide.

How ED is treated

1. Sildenafil: cGMP is broken down by type 5 phosphodiestrerase (PDE_5). Sildenafil (Viagra) inhibits PDE_5 and potentiates the effect of nitric oxide and consequent increase in cGMP.
2. PGE_1 (alprostadil, Caverject, Viridae) potentiates the increase in CAMP, as does VIP (Invicorp).

---

1 Kirby RS. Impotence: diagnosis and management of male erectile dysfunction. *BMJ* 1994;194:694-7
2 Goldstein AMB, Padma-Nathan H. The microarchitecture of the intracavernosal smooth muscle and the cavernosal fibrous skeleton. *J Urol* 1990;144:1144-6
3 Andersson KE, Wagner G. Physiology of penile erection. *Physiol Rev* 1995;75:191-236
4 Burnett AL, Lowenstein CJ, Bredt DS, *et al*. Nitric oxide: a physiologic mediator of penile erection. *Science* 1992;257:401-3
5 Holmes SAV, Kirby RS, Carson C. *Male erectile dysfunction*. Oxford: Health Press, 1997

The cross section of the penis is adapted from A Common Male Problem by Tomlinson J with permission of Pharmica and Upjohn. The diagram of the nerve supply to the penis is adapted from Eardley I, Sethia K, Dean J. *Erectile Dysfunction*. London: Mosby-Wolfe Medical Communications, 1999.

10   Male sexual problems

Alain Gregoire

"My brain? It's my second favourite organ."
Woody Allen, *Sleeper*, 1973

Many men would agree with Woody Allen's implication that
their penis is their favourite organ. This is certainly apparent
to clinicians who deal with human sexuality and who see men
whose penises are not behaving as they should. However,
professionals can become as fixated on this organ as their
patients and forget that it has a multiplicity of connections
within the man's mind and body—and, indeed, outside it.
Our concepts of sexual problems and their assessment and
treatment must reflect this fact if we are to effectively deliver
the help that our patients desperately seek.

It is convenient to consider sexual problems as
dichotomies (organic or psychogenic, primary or secondary,
male or female), but such distinctions are often inaccurate
and unhelpful. The presence of a problem is a subjective
perception influenced by many factors. However, there is no
doubt that for most men sexuality is a highly rated aspect of
their quality of life.

From various studies in the general population and
primary care it seems that 15–20% of men describe some sort
of sexual problem. The proportion of men who actually seek
help is unknown. For many men this is difficult, and their
presentation may be hesitant or disguised in terms of
another complaint. The first and crucial step in managing a
sexual problem is to engage the patient with an interested
and sympathetic attitude. Problems are more likely to occur
in men who are known to their general practitioner because
of physical or mental illness or because of their advancing
age; in such cases an established good relationship will
facilitate communication.

Comorbidity

Given the evolutionary importance of sexual activity, it is not
surprising that it can be adversely affected by almost all forms
of ill health. However, we must remember that we can add to
this sexual morbidity by the treatments we dispense.
Iatrogenic problems are common and are important, if only
because they affect cooperation with treatments.

Physical morbidity
In the general population the perceived association between
physical health and sexual functioning is weak, but in the
clinical setting the relation is more obvious and several
disorders have been linked with sexual problems.

Side effects of treatment
Invasive procedures, such as abdominal, pelvic, or genital
surgery can lead to erectile dysfunction, usually by damage to
peripheral nerves. Postcoital pain may be experienced after
vasectomy because of formation of cysts around the severed
vas.

Many drugs have been associated with male sexual
dysfunctions.

Psychiatric morbidity
All forms of psychiatric disorder can lead to disturbances in
sexuality, either directly, through common effects on the
central nervous system, or indirectly, as a result of social or

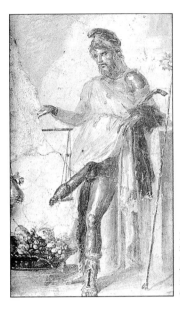

For many men, a properly
functioning penis is fundamental
to their self esteem. (Priapus
weighing his penis—from a fresco
in the Villa dei Vetii, Pompeii, first
century)

Physical causes of male sexual problems

- Peripheral vascular disease
- Diabetes
- Multiple sclerosis
- Spinal injury
- Spinal or brain surgery
- Hormonal or endocrine abnormalities
- Pelvic disease, trauma, or surgery
- Genital abnormality, disease, or surgery
- Consumption of alcohol, tobacco, and
  prescribed and illicit drugs

**Commonly used drugs associated with male sexual
dysfunctions**

- Antihypertensives (such as thiazide diuretics, β blockers)
- Antidepressants (all but a few such as nefazodone and
  mirtazepine)
- Antipsychotics (all, but some are less likely such as olanzapine)
- Anticonvulsants and mood stabilisers (carbamazepine, lithium)
- H$_2$ antagonists (cimetidine)
- Lipid lowering drugs (clofibrate)
- Others—cytotoxic drugs, opiates, digoxin, disulfiram,
  antiandrogens

Managing drug induced side effects

- Delay dosing until after sexual intercourse
- Take "drug holidays" at suitable times, such as
  weekends
- Reduce dose
- Substitute with alternative treatment
- Withdraw drug
- Reduce effects with adjunctive agents

---

psychological changes and drugs' side effects. Depression, anxiety, and schizophrenia are commonly associated with reduced desire and arousal. Mania and hypomania can be accompanied by hypersexuality. However, the assumption, common even among professionals, that people with severe mental illnesses do not need or want satisfying sexual relationships is unfounded.

Recreational drugs

Alcohol is commonly believed to enhance sexuality. Although this is probably true for some men, its inhibitory effects on arousal and its often undesirable behavioural effects are well documented. Increasing levels of consumption are associated with proportionate increases in erectile dysfunction, with 50–80% of alcoholics experiencing impotence. Effects are both immediate and long term, as chronic alcoholics show lowered testosterone concentrations caused by disturbance of the hypothalamic-pituitary axis.

Tobacco consumption also produces immediate and long term effects on erections that are sometimes dramatic.[1] Giving up smoking often leads to improvement. It is surprising that impotence is not cited more often as a persuasive reason for giving up smoking.

Effects of ageing

Ageing is characterised by physiological, pathological, behavioural, and psychosocial changes that can all affect sexual functioning, and it is difficult to disentangle their individual effects. There has been relatively little research into sexuality in old age, but available surveys show that some form of sexual activity usually continues until the end of life. For example, in a sample of people aged 80–102, 62% of the men and 30% of the women were still having sexual intercourse.[2] Clinicians tend to ignore this aspect of the lives of elderly people, who themselves can find sexual problems very difficult to talk about. However, it is wrong to assume that little can be done about problems at this stage in life, as many causes are potentially reversible.[3]

Psychological factors

Research into factors affecting sexual arousal in men has revealed interesting and clinically relevant observations, and the emerging picture is consistent though far from complete.[4]

Anxiety

Anxiety does not have a consistent effect on arousal. It reduces arousal in men with sexual problems but increases arousal in men without. Anxiety related to thoughts of sexual failure have an adverse effect, whereas anxiety associated with novelty or threat is more likely to increase arousal. Men seem to be more susceptible to the effects of anxiety on arousal than women.

Mood

Mood has similarly variable effects. For example, the affective response of men with erectile dysfunction to erotic stimuli is negative, but for men without erectile dysfunction it is positive. Depressed mood causes reduced arousal, thus establishing vicious circles.

Cognitions

Cognitions (thoughts) have a profound effect on sexual response and modulate the effects of mood and anxiety.[5] Patterns of thinking arise from a complex variety of

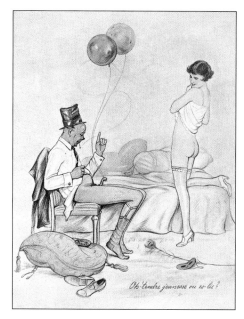

Both alcohol consumption and smoking are associated with erectile dysfunction ("Oh, tender youth, where are you?" from *The Tower of Love* (1920s) by Reunier)

Age related factors leading to sexual dysfunction

- Physical disease—peripheral vascular, diabetic neuropathy
- Psychiatric illness—dementia, depression
- Lack of willing partner, opportunity, or privacy
- Lifestyle factors—smoking, alcohol consumption, physical inactivity, boredom, loneliness

These factors are common and potentially reversible

Sexual changes associated with ageing

- Decreased frequency of activity
- Decreased arousal in response to psychological stimuli
- Decreased tactile sensitivity of penis
- Increased refractory period after orgasm
- Increased rates of erectile dysfunction with age
- Decreased rates of premature ejaculation

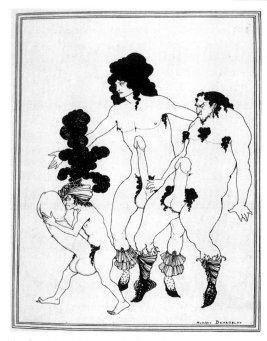

Concern about the size and shape of the penis is a common problem, particularly in young men. (*The Lacedaemonian Ambassadors* (1896) by Aubrey Beardsley)

interacting sources such as a person's cultural, religious, social, educational, and family backgrounds, genetic factors, and past experiences. Understanding these sources in any individual is interesting, but the work of cognitive psychologists shows that changing undesirable cognitions is achieved by helping the person to identify and challenge these thoughts (this is the basis for cognitive therapy, which is used to treat a wide range of mental health problems).

A common example of unhelpful thoughts, particularly in young men, is concern about the size and shape of their penis. Such concerns can lead to considerable difficulties in initiating or maintaining sexual relationships and other sexual problems. Helping men to challenge such concerns by providing information and in other ways is usually very helpful.

Nature of sexual stimulus

Men show more attraction to visual sexual stimuli, whereas women are more attracted to auditory and written material, and in particular stimuli associated with a context of a loving and positive relationship. However, studies of arousal in response to these stimuli show little difference between the sexes.

Relationship

Men with sexual dysfunction are less likely to perceive the quality of their general relationship as relevant to their sexual problems than are their partners or women with sexual problems. Paradoxically, they are more likely to describe improvement in their general relationship in response to successful treatment for sexual problems.

Habituation

Although it is politically controversial, there is considerable evidence that habituation affects responsiveness to sexual stimuli and to partners. Novelty in both increases arousal (the "Coolidge effect") and seems to be more attractive to men than to women.

Dominance and self esteem

Self esteem and social success seem to have a sexually enhancing effect, possibly more so in men than women, and there is evidence that women are more attracted to more powerful or socially dominant men.

Life events

Major events such as bereavements, redundancy, accidents, traumatic experiences, or operations can precipitate changes in sexual behaviour or functioning. Problems that develop in this way can become chronic, particularly if predisposing factors were present. In some cases health professionals can anticipate such problems and have a responsibility to discuss this with their patients—for example, giving information and reassurance about the effects of vasectomy or prostatectomy. Anxieties about the risks of sexual activity after myocardial infarction are common, and advice and reassurance must be given to patients without waiting for them to ask (see previous chapter).

1 Hirshkowitz M, Karacan I, Howell J, Arcasoy M, Williams RL. Nocturnal penile tumescence in cigarette smokers with dysfunction. *Urology* 1992;39:101-7.
2 Bretschneider JG, McCoy NL. Sexual interest and behaviour in healthy 80-102 year olds. *Arch Sex Behav* 1988;17:109-29.
3 Feldman HA, Goldstein I, Hatzichristou DG, Krane RJ, McKinlay JB. Impotence and its medical and psychosocial correlates: results of the Massachusetts male ageing study. *J Urol* 1994;151:54-61.
4 Rosen RC, Leiblum SR. Treatment of sexual disorders in the 1990s: an integrated approach. *J Consult Clin Psychol* 1995;63:877-90.
5 Cranston-Cuebas MA, Barlow DH. Cognitive and affective contributions to sexual functioning. *Annu Rev Sex Res* 1990;1:119-61.

Ways of challenging unhelpful thoughts

- Am I confusing belief with fact?
- Is this belief a helpful way to think about the issue?
- What evidence is there that this belief is true?
- Would other people see things in this way?
- Would I apply the same belief to other people in the same circumstances?
- Am I ignoring evidence that this belief may not be true?
- Am I falling into the trap of overgeneralising or overstating the issue?

Thoughts and erectile dysfunction

	Men without erectile dysfunction	Men with erectile dysfunction
Estimate of quality of own erection	Accurate	Underestimate
Erectile response to distraction	Decrease	Increase
Erectile response to sexual demands	Increase	Decrease

"The Coolidge effect" is so named after the story of Mrs Coolidge, wife of President Coolidge, who on a visit to a farm was impressed by a cockerel's sexual prowess until she was informed that his performance of "a dozen times a day" was with a different hen each time

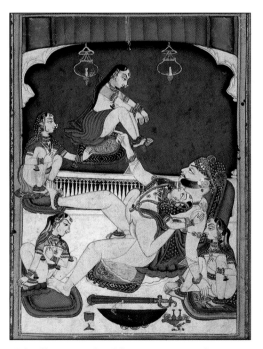

High self esteem and social success seem to enhance a man's sexual function and his attractiveness to women. (A prince enjoying five women from the *Kama Sutra* (1800), from the Rajput School, Kotah, Rajasthan)

The lithograph by Reunier and the painting from the *Kama Sutra* are reproduced with permission of the Bridgeman Art Library.

11 Assessing and managing male sexual problems
Alain Gregoire

Assessing problems

Men are more likely than women to present with and receive treatment for sexual problems. Nevertheless, they usually find them very difficult to talk about, and an initial perception that their problem is being dismissed can considerably delay or prevent their seeking further help. Time spent establishing as clearly as possible the nature of the problem is well spent, as it should lead to more effective treatment and may be therapeutic in itself. Likewise, talking to the partner can reveal a very different picture and can substantially alter management as well as have a therapeutic impact.[1]

Sometimes quite simple interventions—information, reassurance, contraceptive advice, or an opportunity to talk to a member of the primary care team with some basic problem solving or non-directive counselling—can resolve problems that have been a source of considerable distress to patient and partner. Suggesting sources of self help information such as books on sexuality can also be valuable.

When the problem persists despite primary care intervention, further help from other services can be sought, although the provision of services for sexual problems in Britain is variable and rarely enough to meet demand. Optimum assessment and treatment is provided in a multidisciplinary setting, but such clinics are scarce and most patients will be referred to services that have a particular approach. The choice of where to refer a patient will therefore have a critical effect on treatment and, possibly, outcome.

Classification of sexual dysfunction

The accepted diagnostic categories for sexual dysfunction described in ICD-10 (international classification of diseases, 10th revision) and DSM-IV (*Diagnostic and Statistical Manual of Mental Disorders*, fourth revision) do not reflect the reality of sexual dysfunctions in the clinical setting. When these classifications are used it must be remembered that

- Sexual dysfunctions are not all or nothing phenomena but occur on a continuum both in terms of frequency and severity. With our current knowledge, any cut off is inevitably arbitrary
- It is rarely possible to identify cases with a purely organic or purely psychogenic aetiology. Indeed, with our growing knowledge of psychoneuropharmacology and endocrinology, the distinction between organic and psychogenic becomes increasingly blurred
- Comorbidity of sexual dysfunctions is common. For example, nearly half of men with low sexual desire have another sexual dysfunction, and 20% of men with erectile dysfunction have low sexual desire.

In addition to the intrapersonal complexity of sexual problems, the patient's partner and their relationship probably have a more profound effect on sexual health than on any other aspect of health. In up to a third of patients with sexual problems, the partner also has a sexual dysfunction. The interactions between various aspects of sexual problems experienced by a couple are complex, often circular, and rarely reveal simple causal or consequential relationships.

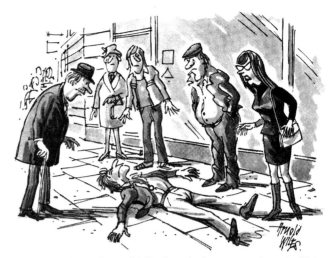

"I'd say loosen his flies but who listens to sex therapists?"

What constitutes a sexual problem?

- Physiological dysfunction
- Altered experiences
- Own perceptions and beliefs
- Partner's perceptions and expectations
- Altered circumstances
- Past experiences

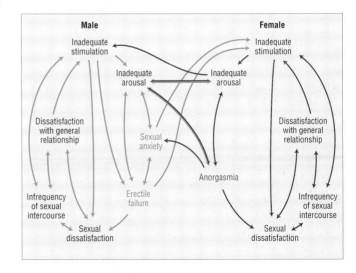

The complex interactions of effects of sexual relationship and general relationship between partners. (Adapted from Gregoire A, Prior JP. *Impotence.* Edinburgh: Churchill Livingstone, 1993)

Inhibited sexual desire

Abnormalities of sexual desire, and indeed sexual desire itself, are difficult to define.[2] The factors considered by clinicians and patients when gauging desire include sexual fantasies, arousal, thoughts, and activity. Given the confusion over the meaning of the concept, it is not surprising that views differ over the term that best describes it. The ICD-10 uses the term sexual desire, and other terms include sexual drive and sexual interest, but "libido" is no longer favoured.

Sexual fantasies, the desire for sexual activity, and distress about the level of desire in a patient and his partner all contribute to the construct of inhibited sexual desire. It is more commonly reported in women than in men (by both women and men) in the general population and in clinic populations. Differences in sexual desire often lead to considerable distress for a couple and can be a source of major conflict in the relationship.

Inhibited sexual desire is often associated with other sexual dysfunctions in the patient or partner. The lifetime prevalence of depression and anxiety disorders is increased. There is a strong association with emotional distance and conflict within a relationship, although it is impossible to determine whether this is cause or consequence from the studies available. Indeed, it is probably meaningless to attempt to do so from population studies given the great individual variability and the very gradual, transactional nature of change in these aspects of relationships.

Characteristic cognitive features have been identified in many cases—for example, the belief that desire does not gradually develop during a sexual encounter but must either be present at the start or does not occur at all, and the belief that subtle feelings such as warmth or tenderness are not sexual and that sexual arousal cannot take place without intense, overtly erotic feelings.

Sexual desire in men can be inhibited by a wide range of physical factors. This can be due to the general effects of illness such as a severe bout of flu or chronic renal failure or to specific effects such as those seen in alcoholism, liver disease, testosterone deficiency, and prolactin secreting pituitary tumours (which may occur in as many as 10% of men presenting with inhibited sexual desire). It is also often a side effect of drugs such as antihypertensives, antidepressants and antipsychotics, anticonvulsants, and cytotoxic agents.

Most studies of outcome indicate that response to psychological intervention for inhibited sexual desire is very poor.[3]

Erectile dysfunction

Erectile dysfunction is dealt with in more detail in the next article of this series. It occurs in 10–15% of men but varies with age, with some degree of dysfunction being experienced by 40% of men at age 40 and by 70% at age 70. In most cases there are both organic and psychological aetiological factors, and assessment and treatment must take account of this.

Various treatments are available, but data on their relative effectiveness and long term outcome are still lacking. Although it is clear that there is no ideal treatment, there is usually one that is both effective and acceptable to the man and his partner. Sildenafil represents an important advance but seems to be a victim of its own success, with concerns about costs leading to limitations on prescription as well as there being evidence of misuse.[4]

Premature ejaculation

Premature ejaculation is an inability to control ejaculation sufficiently to permit both partners to enjoy sexual

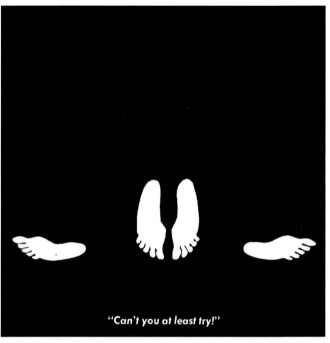

"Can't you at least try!"

Differences in sexual desire often lead to considerable distress for a couple and can be a source of major conflict in the relationship

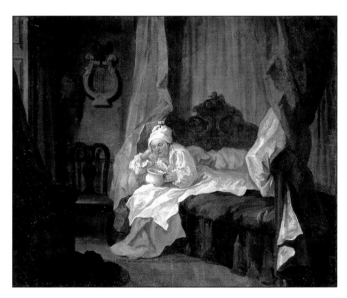

Sexual desire can be inhibited by physical factors such as the effects of illness. (*Francis Matthew Schutz in his Bed* (circa 1755-60) by William Hogarth)

"A hard man is good to find"   Mae West

Treatments for erectile impotence

- Simple measures—education, advice, self help books
- Psychological—therapy for couples or for single men individually or in groups
- Oral drugs—sildenafil
- Topical vasodilators
- Intracavernosal drugs—prostaglandin E_1
- Vacuum devices
- Prosthetic implants
- Surgery for venous leakage

intercourse. This may result in ejaculation shortly after penetration or, in severe cases, before penetration.

Sometimes the true problem is an erectile difficulty that necessitates prolonged stimulation in order to achieve adequate erection, and there is therefore an apparently short period before ejaculation. About 20% of men complain of premature ejaculation, and in the vast majority of cases there is no evidence of any physical underlying cause. Premature ejaculation is commoner in younger men, and it is likely that there is a process of learning to control ejaculation with increasing sexual experience. Anxiety undoubtedly plays an important role in hastening ejaculation in some men.

Psychological interventions are aimed at reducing performance anxiety and improving ejaculatory control— such as by the "pause and squeeze" technique. Reported success rates are conflicting, and long term follow up suggests that benefits are not maintained.[5]

Drug treatment with specific serotonin reuptake inhibitor antidepressants such as sertraline 50 mg daily are effective in delaying ejaculation and improving sexual satisfaction in patient and partner. Recent studies indicate that intermittent use can be as effective as continuous use, and this should reduce the rates of undesirable side effects such as nausea and decreased desire.

Retarded and absent ejaculation

Retrograde, absent, or retarded ejaculation caused by drug side effects are seen fairly frequently in clinic populations, although many sufferers do not spontaneously complain but simply stop their medication. Common causes include antidepressant and antipsychotic drugs as well as prostatectomy. Cases not associated with these obvious causes are rare.

Psychological treatment focuses on reducing anxiety and increasing arousal. Increased genital stimulation is important, and patients sometimes need encouragement and "permission" to pursue this, including using aids such as a vibrator. One successful option for treating antidepressant induced anorgasmia is the adjunctive use of cyproheptadine (2–16 mg) before sexual intercourse. However, this is a serotonin antagonist and has been reported to cause relapse of the depression in some cases.

Dyspareunia

Genital pain before, during, or after intercourse is rare in men, occurring in about 1% of clinic samples. The cause can be physical, such as genital infection, phimosis, and prostatitis, or psychological. There are at present no outcome studies of psychological treatments for this distressing problem.

The cartoon "I'd loosen his flies. . ." is reproduced with permission of Punch Publications. The painting by Hogarth is reproduced with permission of the Bridgeman Art Library. The cartoon "Can't you at least try?" is by Neville Spearman.

1 Ackerman MD, Carey MP. Psychology's role in the assessment of erectile dysfunction: historical precedents, current knowledge and methods. *J Consult Clin Psychol* 1995;63:862-76.
2 Gayle Beck J. Hypoactive sexual desire disorder: an overview. *J Consult Clin Psychol* 1995;63:915-27.
3 Hawton K. Treatment of sexual dysfunctions by sex therapy and other approaches. *Br J Psychiatry* 1995;167:307-14.
4 Gregoire A. Viagra: on release. *BMJ* 1998;317:759-60.
5 Rosen RC, Leiblum SR. Treatment of sexual disorders in the 1990s: an integrated approach. *J Consult Clin Psychol* 1995;63:877-90.

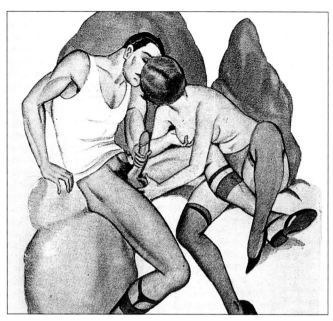

The "pause and squeeze" technique can be used to try to improve ejaculatory control. (Illustration for *The Book of Lust* (1920-30) by Pierre Lacombière)

Sources of further help for patients*

Relate—Local availability of services and waiting lists vary across the country. A fee is charged. Will usually see people individually but prefer to see couples together. Offer marital as well as sexual counselling

Family planning clinics—Sometimes also offer psychosexual counselling services

Brook advisory centres—Usually provide advice and sexual counselling. Particularly suitable for young adults

Urology clinics—Usually assess only organic causes and provide physical treatments, mainly for erectile dysfunction

Psychiatry departments—Now rarely do any work with sexual problems as priority is given to serious mental illness. Some psychiatry departments have special clinics for sexual problems

Sexual dysfunction clinics—The better clinics are multidisciplinary and can assess both psychological and organic aspects of a problem and can provide psychological and physical treatments. These clinics probably offer the best service, but there are few of them and waiting lists tend to be long

*List of clinics available from the honorary secretary, British Association of Sexual and Marital Therapy, PO Box 62, Sheffield S10 3TS

Recommended further reading

• Bancroft J. *Human sexuality and its problems.* 2nd ed. Edinburgh: Churchill Livingstone, 1989
  Although this book is now a little old and in need of revision in some areas (such as management of erectile dysfunction), it remains one of the best comprehensive textbooks in the subject
• Gregoire A, Prior JP. *Impotence: an integrated approach to clinical practice.* Edinburgh: Churchill Livingstone, 1993
  A comprehensive textbook covering psychological and physical aspects of erectile disorders and their management
• Baldwin D, Thomas S. *Depression and sexual function.* London: Martin Dunitz, 1996
  Available from Bristol Myers Squibb Pharmaceuticals

12 Erectile dysfunction
Wallace Dinsmore, Christine Evans

Treatment of erectile dysfunction is initiated after taking a patient's history and examination (see previous articles), and possibly investigation.

Medical management

In highly selected patients with a clear psychological problem, psychotherapy or sex and couple therapy can be used, but these are time consuming and available to only a small number of patients. Nevertheless, it is essential to treat the whole person and not just his penis. Counselling, alone or separately from sensate focus techniques[1] should be considered as options. Erectile dysfunction is of a largely psychological nature in a third of patients, in a third it is largely physical and the remaining third have both physical and psychological factors.

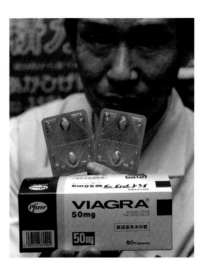

Oral treatment

Sildenafil The first line of treatment for erectile dysfunction with most practitioners at the time of writing is oral sildenafil. Despite much exaggeration of its seemingly magical powers, it is a very significant advance in management with an overall success rate of 69%.[2] Initial reports suggest an effective response of 88% in those who have psychogenic causes and the treatment may have its effect by breaking the failure cycle. It seems to be well tolerated and particularly effective in men with post traumatic spinal cord injury, who have partial preservation of erectile function.[3] In diabetics, the success rate is lower, averaging about 50% of those treated.

Sildenafil is marketed as tablets of 25, 50 and 100 mgs. The optimum dose is found by starting at 50 mg and titrating upwards or downwards. The most effective dose seems to be 50–100 mg. Doses greater than 100 mg do not appear to improve the response, although the side effects are more common. These are headache (16%), flushing (10%), dyspepsia (7%) nasal congestion (4%) and transient green/blue tingeing of vision in 3% with higher doses.[2] Priapism has not been recorded. Total contraindications are concurrent use of sildenafil with nitrates used for angina or hypertension.[4]

The drug needs to be taken an hour (or $1\frac{1}{2}$ hours after a meal), before sexual activity and does not work unless there is physical or mental sexual stimulation, a fact which needs to be spelled out carefully to some patients (and their partners).

Yohimbine is not licensed but has been used for many decades at a dosage of 5–15 mg daily. Many specialists believe its effects to be largely placebo related.

Injection treatment

Alprostadil (prostaglandin E_1) was given a product licence in 1994 and is supplied in 5, 10, and 20 μg doses. Patients are usually started on a small dose in the clinic but are advised that the injection may be more effective in a more relaxed atmosphere at home. Lower doses are more likely to be effective in counteracting neurological disease.

Investigation of erectile dysfunction

Mandatory
- Blood pressure
- Glucose (blood or urine)

If reduced sex drive
- Testosterone—total, serum hormone binding globulin (SHBG), and free androgen index (FAI)
- Follicle stimulating hormone (FSH)
- Luteinising hormone (LH)
- Prolactin—especially for reduced sex drive in a younger man

Other possible investigations
- Nocturnal erection testing by "snap gauge" or Rigiscan
- Vascular function
  Doppler colour ultrasound
  Response to injected drugs
  Arteriography

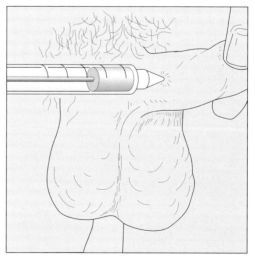

Intracavernosal injection of alprostadil

Possible side effects of intracavernosal injection include bruising, pain, priapism, and fibrosis

Papaverine was introduced in the early 1980s as the first effective intracavernosal injection treatment for erectile dysfunction. Given in doses of 7.5–90 mg, initially alone and later with phentolamine as a synergist in the ratio of 30:1, these treatments did not have a product licence but they were effective, cheap, and easy to use, although they had a high incidence (up to 25%) of prolonged erection.

Triple therapy (a combination of papaverine, phentolamine, and alprostadil) is used for patients in whom individual drugs have failed. Treatment usually starts at a dose of papaverine 30 mg, phentolamine 1 mg, and alprostadil 20 µg.

Vasoactive intestinal polypeptide (VIP), 0.025 mg in combination with phentolamine (1 mg or 2 mg), has recently received a licence, and there have been early reports of success from trials.

Consent forms for treatment may be used, especially if unlicensed preparations are being prescribed. All these treatments are intracavernosal and should be initiated under careful medical supervision. Initial doses for all compounds are usually low because of the risk of priapism (an erection lasting longer than 4-6 hours). As this may occur with intracavernosal injections, it is essential that practitioners familiarise themselves with the treatment of priapism (see box).

Intraurethral treatment
If sildenafil does not work the medicated urethral system for erection (MUSE) can be tried. It is a pellet of prostaglandin (in doses of 125, 250, 500, or 1000 µg) which is placed in the urethra through the meatus and produces an erection after about 15 minutes. This treatment is a popular choice for both patients and physicians because of its ease of use, but, in common with other prostaglandin treatments, it has a relatively high incidence of penile pain and also appears to have a low efficacy which may make patients less willing to continue the treatment.

Hormonal treatment
Testosterone is usually ineffective in treating erectile dysfunction in patients with normal serum testosterone concentrations and may exacerbate the problem by increasing a patient's sexual drive without improving his ability to perform. It may be given orally but is usually given as an intramuscular depot injection at intervals of 3–4 weeks, by daily patches, or by implants every six months. Great care should be exercised in patients with possible carcinoma of the prostate, and levels of prostate specific antigen (PSA) should be checked initially and every six months.

Ethical considerations
Some clinics insist on seeing both members of a couple before starting treatment, but many clinics see only the male partner and are therefore totally reliant on his history. However, many patients are not in a relationship and are afraid to embark on one because of fear of erectile failure. The confidence gained by the certainty of obtaining an erection enables a proportion of this group (whether their problem is psychological or physical) to initiate a relationship, and many patients will have a resumption of normal erectile function.

Misuse of these drugs is a consideration. There are isolated reports of the use of intracavernosal injections in association with prostitution and anecdotal reports of their use in sex shows, and this may become a big problem with oral sildenafil. After a drug is prescribed there is clearly no possibility of monitoring its use. It is impossible to check for

---

Treatment of priapism

If a man has an artificial erection that lasts more than 4 hours it must be treated as an emergency
The longer that it is left the more likely it is that he will have, at best, fibrosis or, at worst, gangrene of the corpora

Management
1 Aspirate 50 ml of blood from each corpus through a 19 gauge butterfly needle into a 50 ml syringe with a Luer lock
2 If penis becomes flaccid and then rigid again open an ampoule of phenylephrine* 10 mg in 1 ml, take out 0.2 ml (2 mg), and dilute in 10 ml of normal saline
3 Inject 1 ml (200 µg) of phenylephrine solution through the same butterfly needle and aspirate, if necessary, a couple of minutes later. Repeat this every 5-10 minutes until a total of 5 ml (1 mg) of solution has been injected
   Alternatively, a 20 µg/ml solution of adrenaline can be used, with further aspiration
   The maximum dose of phenylephrine should be 1 mg, and the maximum dose of adrenaline should be 100 µg (5 ml)
4 Metaraminol* (1 mg in 50 ml saline) can be substituted, given slowly in 5 ml doses every 15 minutes. This should not be used in patients taking monoamine oxidase inhibitors
5 On removing the needle, get the patient to press firmly for 5 minutes to prevent massive bruising
6 If none of the above works urologists should be called in

The blood pressure and pulse should be closely monitored, especially with hypertensive or atherosclerotic patients and those taking monoamine oxidase inhibitors. For such patients, facilities should be available to manage a potential hypertensive crisis, which may, rarely, be fatal

*A vasoconstrictor sympathomimetic

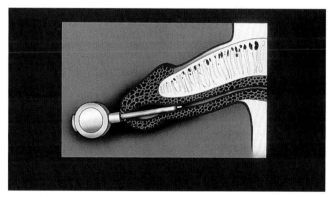

MUSE (alprostadil)

Hormonal treatment for erectile dysfunction
- Testosterone should be used (usually intramuscularly) only for patients with low testosterone levels (free or total)
- Patients should be monitored for possible carcinoma of the prostate, for example, by six monthly checks of prostatic specific antigen (PSA) levels

paedophile and other sexual offences, and patients in these groups may receive help to restore erectile function, with obvious medicolegal implications.

The treatment of homosexual men may be a reflection of an individual doctor's prejudices. As a patient's history is the only evidence available, it would clearly be discriminatory not to treat men who have male partners. Some doctors prefer not to, or refuse to, treat patients who are infected with HIV, but, unless there is uniform testing of all patients, this information is usually available only if the patient volunteers it.

Erectile problems are common in men infected with HIV, and some clinics are now treating infected patients, who are usually in long term relationships. Before treatment, both partners are usually counselled about the risks involved and are asked to give signed agreement to treatment. Again, as in heterosexual relationships, injections may be used in a commercial situation. The occurrence of HIV being knowingly transmitted after treatment to restore erectile function is extremely rare, and there have been no reported cases in the United Kingdom.

Vacuum devices

There are many vacuum devices, either manual or battery operated, currently available for treating erectile dysfunction. The penis placed in a plastic tube, and venous blood is drawn into it by suction. Once it is erect, a rubber constriction ring is placed at its base to prevent detumescence. These devices are generally safe, but the erection should not be maintained for more than 30 minutes as the penis may become cold and painful because of the constriction. Vacuum devices are the preferred option for patients who are afraid of injections or in whom injections have not been successful. They cost from £100 to £300 and are usually supported by manufacturers' helplines and money back guarantees.

Surgical management

Surgery for venous leakage and microvascular techniques for revascularisation of the corpora are rarely done, and the results are not good. The only surgical treatment of any value is inserting a penile prosthesis. Since their advent in the mid-1970s, prostheses have developed considerably from poorly concealed, low cost, trimmable silastic rods to ones made of silicone outside a metal core and self contained, inflatable cylinders. Inflatable devices are either two part prostheses with a combined reservoir and pump that sits in the scrotum or three piece models in which the pump alone sits in the scrotum and the reservoir lies in the lower abdominal wall.

Indications for use of prostheses have changed with the development of intracorporeal injections, vacuum devices, and oral preparations. Patients commonly needing surgery are those who have had pelvic surgery or who have diabetes or atherosclerosis. Prostheses are also useful in patients impotent with Peyronie's disease (which seems to be getting commoner) as they correct the deformity as well as the impotence.

Cost apart, the choice of prosthesis is up to the patient. The semi-rigid cylinders do stick out and are therefore not suitable for younger men with children in the house, those participating in swimming and sporting events, and naturists. The cost of an inflatable prosthesis is not countenanced by some NHS trusts, but persuasion may be possible in a particularly deserving case such as a young diabetic patient impotent through no fault of his own and whose marriage is at risk.

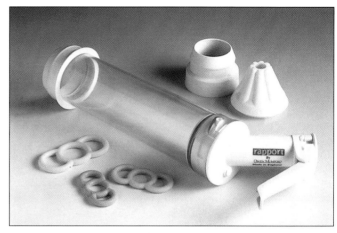

Vacuum pump and constriction rings

Indications for a penile prosthesis

Organic impotence
- Problems with intracavernosal drugs and external devices (unwilling to consider them, failure to respond to them, unable to continue with them)
- Penile fibrosis from injection
- Peyronie's disease with impotence
- Damage after priapism

Psychological impotence
- After all other treatments have failed

Costs of prostheses*

Semi-rigid malleable	£650–720
Inflatable two piece	£1995–2300
Inflatable three piece	£2700–3700

*Prices for 1998 excluding VAT

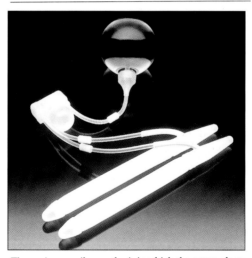

Three piece penile prosthesis in which the pump alone sits in the scrotum and the reservoir lies in the lower abdominal wall

Preoperative counselling about a penile prosthesis

Counsel patient, with partner, that
- The glans will not be filled
- The result will be adequate for vaginal penetration
- There is a small (2–5%) incidence of infection
- The penis will be colder
- Ejaculation will still be possible
- The only solution to a failed operation is a replacement prosthesis
- A prosthesis is not as good as the original

Operative procedure

The operation is done under regional or general anaesthesia. Circumcision is often necessary with many semi-rigid prostheses, so this should be done initially.

The corpora are exposed and opened through an incision large enough to insert a Hegars dilator and are dilated full length from just inside the glans to the ischium, compressing the normal corpora. This may be difficult with fibrotic penises, after priapism, or with Peyronie's plaques. With multipart prostheses, all components are filled with saline and the tubing connected, the pump is placed in the most dependent part of the scrotum, and the reservoir is put under the rectus sheath.

Postoperative management

Pain relief must be provided as the operation is painful.

Antibiotics—A broad spectrum antibiotic should be taken orally for a week after the operation.

Voiding—If there are difficulties with voiding, use clean intermittent catheterisation.

Postoperative use—Semi-rigid prostheses may be used after four weeks. Patients can be taught how to pump up an inflatable prosthesis after four to six weeks.

Postoperative problems

Infection occurs in 1–10% of cases, depending on the difficulty of the procedure. Repeat operations are more prone to infection. It is usually necessary to remove the infected part or complete prosthesis, and, although difficult, it is possible to replace it six months later.

Erosion is usually due to infection or to an unsuspected breach of the urethra at surgery.

Glans ischaemia occurs with vascular compression or damage.

Supersonic transport (SST) deformity (also known as Concorde deformity) with glans droop may be unsightly but may not matter if there is an additional glandular erection.

Mechanical problems are now uncommon. If they occur the part should be replaced.

Prognosis

Penile prostheses give acceptable results. In many large series over 80% of patients and their partners were satisfied with the results. In those with Peyronie's disorder, a prosthesis straightened the penises of 70%. There is no real age limit for the operation, but a prosthesis should not be inserted unless it is going to be used.

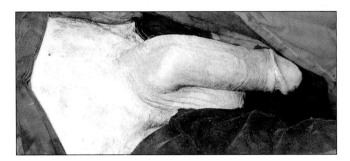

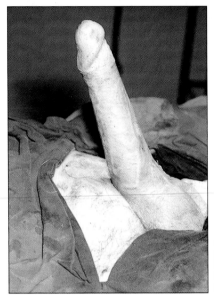

Appearance of a penis after insertion of an inflatable prosthesis, with the device deflated (top) and inflated (left)

1 Masters WH, Johnson VE, and Kolodny RC. *Human sexuality* New York: Harper Collins, 5th ed, pp 358–68, 1995.
2 *Sildenafil for erectile dysfunction* Drug and Therapeutics Bulletin **36** 81–84 (Nov 1998).
3 Derry F, Glass C, Dinsmore WW et al. Sildenafil (Viagra): a double-blind, placebo controlled, single dose, two way cross over study in men with erectile dysfunction caused by traumatic spinal cord injury. *J Neurol Sci* 1997; **150**(suppl):S134(abstract 2-52-10).
4 Morales A, Gingell C, Wicker PA, Osterloh IH. Clinical safety of oral sildenafil citrate (Viagra) in the treatment of erectile dysfunction *Int J Impot Res* 1998;**10**:69–74.

The picture of Viagra is produced with permission of *Associated Press.*

13   Homosexual men and women

Robin Bell

The range of sexual dysfunctions encoutered in gay men and lesbians is the same as that found in men and women in general, and the skills needed to help them are the same. That said, there are areas of concern, both for patients and doctors, that merit particular consideration.

People may encounter problems when they become aware of their homosexual orientation and try to match it to their view of an ideal self. If this occurs in adolescence it may be useful to offer counselling to help with the readjustment in life that may be required. However tolerant our society may become, being openly gay still has major implications for future carerr and family life. Help at this time can include (for men especially) information about safer sex, since sexual exploration may present a greater risk of exposure to HIV.

Although many gay men and lesbians are aware of their orientation from their earliest sexual thoughts, a sizeable minority do not discover their orientation until later in life, perhaps in a failing marriage and with the responsibilities of parenthood. These people require careful and compassionate counselling. Some choose to remain married, and the couple may need help to reorganise the basis of their heterosexual relationship. The counsellor must be seen to be completely impartial and not encourage any particular outcome.

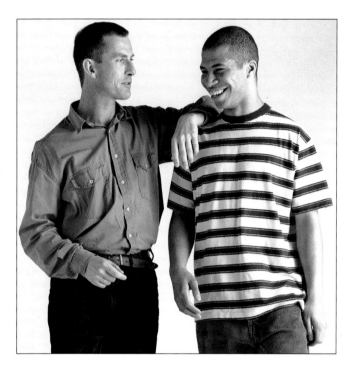

Avoiding prejudice

Presumptions—When counselling gay people about sex, it is important not to have preconceived ideas about their sexual repertoire. Perhaps as many as a third of gay men choose not to practise penetrative anal sex on a regular basis,[1] and the traditional division of gay men into "active" and "passive" is not born out by experience—most gay men who do have anal sex will play either role. The assumption that the passive partner is somehow less "male" or less "aggressive" is also largely a myth. Similarly, in lesbian sex either partner can be psychologically "active" regardless of whether sex play includes penetration with a dildo.

Disapproval—The days when physicians would try to impose their own moral standards on their patients should be long past. In individual clinicians are aware that they are uncomfortable with the issues of gay sex and relationships then they should refer thte patient on to somebody else. It is difficult to focus on the relevant clinical issues if you are having to concentrate on your own discomfort and trying not to express it.

Inaccurate advice—It is unwise to advise patients on subjects that they may know more about than you do, and if anal sex is not something that you know much about it is better to admist this rather than offer inaccurate or misleading advice. Local genitourinary medicine clinics should be aware of what services are available locally and which are considered as "gay friendly" and can be used as a source of reference.

Patients' reticence—Even if a doctor is comfortable with homosexual patients it does not follow that such patients are comfortable with the doctor. Gay men face practical problems, such as a future application for life insurance, which mean that some patients will not wish to disclose their sexual orientation to their general practitioner, no matter how sympathetic and confidential.

Counselling gay men and women

- Be honest with yourself; if you are uncomfortable with gay people refer the patient to someone else
- If an adolescent is confused about his or her sexuality try to help the patient to adjust
- Do not have preconceived ideas
- Take the opportunity to discuss safe sex with gay men
- A married man or woman might benefit from couples counselling
- Sexual orientation is not always fixed. Some people change their mind

---

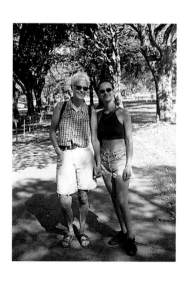

Sexual activities

It is unclear what proportion of men and women have same sex experiences in their lives. Studies have been fraught with methodological errors and with researchers trying to confirm methodological errors and with researchers trying to confirm their own preconceptions. Recently, the national survey of sexual attitudes and lifestyles estimated that 1% to 6% of the male population had had such experiences, depending on how homosexuality was defined.[2] These values are lower than many other estimates, probably because of the method of the study.

Gay men and lesbians have as wide a range of sexual lifestyles as does the general community. Some homosexuals live in a stable partnership and never have sex elsewhere. Others have a strong, committed relationship but with an open acknowledgment that one or both partners also have sexual liaisons elsewhere. Infidelity in a supposedly closed relationship is probably just as common as among heroesexuals. Single gay men have a reputation for having many sexual partners, and in urban communities the opportunities for this are widespread. Casual or anonymous sex can provide sexual gratification without the complications of a relationship.

Sexual dysfunctions should be assessed objectively without a moral stance being taken on the manner in which sexual expression is likely to occur.[3] Similarly, casual sex can be the reason for patients, male or female, to seek help, realising that although they are sexually fulfilled, they are "missing out" on the emotional aspects that can be associated with sex as part of a relationship. There can also be considerable distress for those who find it difficult to establish same sex relationships that could progress to become sexual and committed.

Spectrum of activity

Gay men—Anal sex remains a taboo subject even for many professional sexual discussions; however, it is widely practised in most communities. Sexual activity is protean in all groups, and gay men are no different in this with much research having been done into their behaviour. Mutual masturbation, oral sex, and anal sex can be considered core activities, although many gay men do not practise anal sex at all. In recent years however, there has been an increase in anal eroticism involving rimming (tongue/anus contact), inserting foreign bodies (butt plugs, dildos) and water sports (urination). Some couples may choose more vigorous forms of penetration such as fisting, in which the hand and part of the forearm is introduced into the rectum.

Lesbians—There has been little authoritative research into lesian sexual life and activities, in contrast with the very large amount into male homosexuals, which was accelerated by the appearance of AIDS. However, one study found that the order of frequency of different types of sexual activity among lesbians was mutual masturbation, oral sex (cunnilingus) and body rubbing (which was more common among black women). The use of dildos and fisting (see vocabulary) is probably no more common than in heterosexual couples.

Terminology

Once they have sought help, gay men and women are often less reticent in discussing at length and in detail specific sexual acts. It is therefore useful for a doctor to be forearmed with a basic vocabulary of gay sex, although many men and women who perform these activities will lack the words to describe them, and few people of any orientation are likely to have all the activites in their personal behavioural repertoire.

The terms "active" and "passive" are best avoided if a doctor needs to determine the content of a sexual act, such as

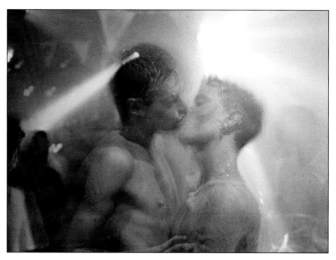

Casual or anonymous sex can provide sexual gratification without the complications of a relationship

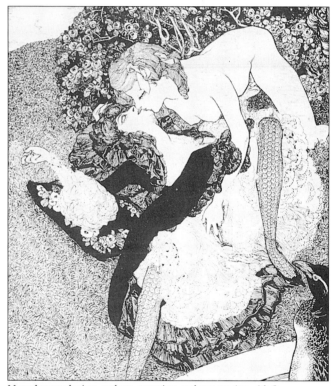

Mutual masturbation, oral sex, caressing, and penetration with fingers or sex toys can be considered as core activities of lesbian sex. ("Anything is possible!" from *La Grenouillère* (1907) by Franz von Bayros)

A gay sexual vocabulary

B/D—Bondage and domination. The use of power play, but not pain, for sexual pleasure

Back room—That part of a sleaze bar (see below) where sex can take place

Cottaging—The use of public toilets as a venue for meeting sexual partners

Cruising—To be actively looking for a sexual partner

Fisting—The insertion of a whole hand into the rectum or vagina for sexual stimulation

Rimming—Oro-anal contact for sexual stimulation

Sleaze bar—A bar or pub where sex can be performed on the premises

S/M—Sadomasochism, the use of pain in consensual sexual acts

Vanilla—Sex that does not extend beyond affection, mutual masturbation, and oral and anal sex. This is the commonest mode of gay sexual expression

Water sports—Urination as a sexual pleasure

when considering the risks of sexually transmitted disease. The doctor's concerns are anatomical placement and not the psychological roles implied by these words. Most gay men will not fit exclusely into either of the roles implied by the old fashioned heterosexual model, and if the words are applied to oral sex great confusion may result. Gay male oral sex includes two sexual acts, fellation and irrumation—cock sucking and face fucking respectively—depending on whether it is the mouth sucking or the penis thrusting that is the main act. In both cases there is a penis in the mouth, but the "active" partner differs. When it is necessary to determine who did what, it is easier to talk about insertive and receptive partners to avoid confusion.

Facts and figures

- Two thirds of gay men have anal sex
- Ten per cent of heterosexual couples regularly have anal sex
- The estimate that 6% of the male population are gay may be an understatement
- No one knows how common sexual problems are in this group
- Their presentation varies widely from clinic to clinic
- Erectile dysfunction is increasingly seen in men infected with HIV
- Retarded ejaculation is common
- Piles and anal fissures are no more common in gay men than in the general population
- Vaginismus, anorgbasmia, and low sex drive occur in lesbians as in heterosexual women

Problems

Erectile dysfunction is being seen increasingly, usually of an organi type, in those with late stage HIV infection, although whether this is an effect of the virus or of the antivial drugs is not yet clear.

Retarded ejaculation is common in gay men and may be related to fears of contagion induced by the "safer sex" campaigns.

Piles caused by dilation of an anal venous plexus are no more common in those having receptive anal sex, and are usually caused by straining at stool.

Anal fissures usually arise from constipation rather than receptive anal sex. However, if they are a sexual problem they generally respond to the use of an anal dilator. The medical St Mark's type is readily available, and the self retaining version is sold as a sex toy called a "butt plug." The smallest size works well if left in situ for several hours each evening. A topical anaesthetic (such as EMLA cream) may be used on the first few occastions, until healing is under way.

Female sexual problems—Like heterosexual women, lesbians can suffer from vaginismus, primary or secondary, and from anorgasmia and low sexual drive (see earlier chapters by Butcher).

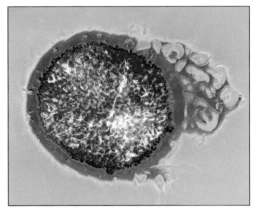

Infection with *Neisseria gonorrhoeae* can occur through oral sex as well as vaginal and anal sex

Infections associated with homosexual activity

- Sexually transmitted diseases are common in all gay people with a high number of different partners
- Their management is the same as in the heterosexual community
- The transmission of infection through vaginal and anal intercourse is no different, apart from HIV
- Hepatitis A and *Giardia* are spread through oro-anal contact
- The greater incidence of hepatitis B is an indicator of a large number of partners, not of specific sexual practices

Infections

Sexually transmitted diseases are common in people with many sexual partners, which includes some homosexual men. The ease of transmission of most sexual infections is similar for vaginal and anal sex, with the exception of HIV, which is much more easily spread by anal sex. Strong condoms greatly reduce this risk. Oral sex, while a recognised route of transmission, is considered to be relatively safe for HIV, but it is a common means of acquiring gonorrhoea and non-specific urethritis. Lesbians are considered a low risk group for HIV infection.

Faeco-oral spread of pathogens such as *Giardia* and hepatitis A are well recorded from oro-anal sexual contact. Minor episodes of diarrhoea may be related to faecal exposure, and are often self limiting. If they persist, stool culture will usually pick up any bacterial cause, and if the culture is negative it is better to treat for presumed giardiasis than do extensive investigations to attempt to prove the diagnosis.´

Hepatitis B, though commoner in gay men, has not been shown to be spread by specific sexual practices and may simply be a marker of exposure to a greater number of sexual partners. The orthodox sexually transmitted diseases are managed as in the heterosexual community, although contact tracing for gay men with non-specific urethritis is less important given the rarity (2%) of chlamydia as a causative agent in gay men.

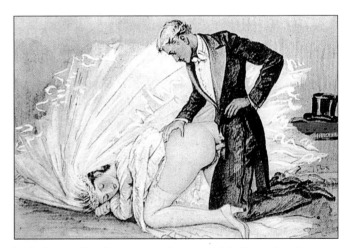

In absolute numbers there are more heterosexuals having anal sex in Britain than there are gay men. (Illustration (possibly by Paul-Emile Bécat) for *An Up-to-date Young Lady* (1920s) by Helena Varley)

Immunisation against hepatitis A and B is recommended by the Department of Health for all men with male sexual contacts.

Anal sex

About a third of heterosexual couples in Britain are thought to use anal sex as an occasional method of sexual expression, with about 10% using it as a preferred or regular method.[2] Perhaps two thirds of gay men practise anal sex as a regular part of their sexual repertoire. This means that, in absolute numbers, there are more heterosexuals having anal sex than there are gay men. There are little published data on how many heterosexual men would like their anus to be sexually stimulated in a heterosexual relationship. Anecdotally, it is a substantial number. What data we do have almost all relate to penetrative sexual acts, and the superficial contact of the anal ring with fingers or the tongue is even less well documented but may be assumed to be a common sexual activity for men of all sexual orientations.

Anatomy of the anus

The nerve supply to the anal margin is the same as that to the genitalia, coming from S4, and the pectinate line roughly marks the division between sensitivity to touch and temperature externally and perception of little more than stretch internally. The external and sphincter is made of striated muscle and can be brought under voluntary control, whereas the internal sphincter, which is a thickening of the intrinsic muscle layer of the gut, is made of smooth muscle and is autonomic, opening in response to stretch stimuli.

Advice for patients

- Check that the patient really wants to try anal sex and is not being pressured by a partner
- Anal relaxation is better than pushing harder
- Reinforce the use of condoms with water based lubrication as a protection against HIV
- Give instructions for anal dilatation and relaxation exercises

Anal dilatations and relaxation exercises

- Do these exercises on your own until you are confident you can accommodate a penis
- Start doing exercises in bed lying on a towel or lying on your back in a warm bath
- Raise your knees towards your chest
- Explore the perianal area with a finger covered in lubrication. Petroleum jelly is a good choice at this stage, but it must be substituted with a water based lubricant before intercourse with a condom is attempted
- Gentle pressure with a finger moving a circle round the anus will relax the phincter enough to be able to insert one digit
- Once the finger can be comfortably accommodated, begin to stretch the sphincter with circling motions inside the anus
- After several sessions, it will be possible to insert another finger and to continue
- Further dilation by relaxation, not stretching, can be achieved by the use of an anal dilator of the St Mark's type or a self retaining "butt plug" left in situ on a regular basis.

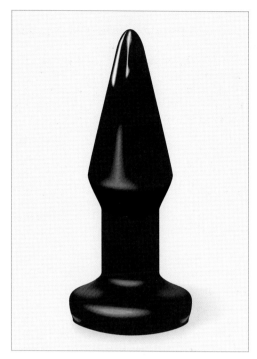

A self retaining "butt plug," which can be used in anal dilatation exercises or simply as a sex toy

1 Coxon A. *Between the sheets*. London: Cassell, 1996.
2 Wellings K, Field J, Johnson N, Wadsworth J. *Sexual behaviour in Britain. The national survey of sexual attitudes and lifestyles*. London: Penguin Books, 1994.
3 General Medical Council. *Good medical practice*. London: GMC, 1998.

The picture of the male gay couple is by Fly Design Consultants and reproduced with permission of the Terrence Higgins Trust. The picture of gay men in a night club is by Nathan Cox and reproduced with permission of Gaze International. The picture of the lesbian couple is reproduced with permission of Gaze International. The electron micrograph of gonorrhoea bacterium is by A B Dowsett and reproduced with permission of Science Photo Library.

14 Sexual problems of disabled patients

Clive Glass, Bakulesh Soni

Almost 4% of the UK population have some form of physical, sensory, or intellectual impairment—almost 2.5 million people. Many of these disabling conditions can produce sexual problems of desire, arousal, orgasm, or sexual pain in men and women. Sexual difficulties may arise from direct trauma to the genital area (due to either accident or disease), damage to the nervous system (such as spinal cord injury), or as an indirect consequence of a non-sexual illness (cancer of any organ may not directly affect sexual abilities but can cause fatigue and reduce the desire or ability to engage in sexual activity).

The two main points for consideration are how disabling conditions affect sexual function and behaviour and which sexual difficulties most commonly arise.

Effects of disability on sexual function

Women who undergo radical mastectomy or a disfiguring trauma often report concerns about their femininity and self image such as feelings of lowered self worth or the fear that men will find them less attractive. Similarly, young men with erectile dysfunction often avoid meeting potential partners because of their embarrassment over their inability to perform.

"Sexuality" describes how people express their view of what is sexual. That awareness is the result of all the physical, emotional, intellectual, and social factors that have influenced their development up to that point in their life. Defining sexuality as wider than just physical function is particularly important for people with disabilities. A person who is not able to use part of his or her body still has an equal right to full sexual expression.

Congenital or acquired disability

Congenital or birth impairments often affect all aspects of sexual development, and lack of privacy and independence in daily living means adolescents often miss out on normal sexual experiences. In contrast, an acquired disability may have different implications depending on when it happened. Impairments early in life often produce low social and sexual confidence, whereas patients who become disabled in adulthood are much more aware of what has actually been lost. While the degree of adjustment to either form of impairment may be no different, the process of adjustment is different. How people view their disability and who they see as responsible for managing the effects of the condition greatly influences their ability to cope.

Hidden impairment

Patients with an impairment that is hidden from others but which affects continence or sexual function often find the situation unbearable. People with spina bifida and perineal paraplegia often walk without apparent difficulty but experience problems with sexual function and with controlling their bladder and bowel. The unpredictability of control often leads them to avoid social mixing, therefore increasing their isolation. People with disabilities often present with low self confidence and a poor body image, and so clinicians should not confuse the severity of a condition with the severity of its impact on the patient.

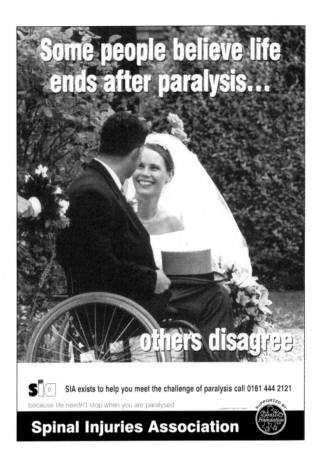

Some people believe life ends after paralysis... others disagree

SIA exists to help you meet the challenge of paralysis call 0181 444 2121

because life needn't stop when you are paralysed

Spinal Injuries Association

Key questions in cases of disability

Present condition
- Has the person congenital or acquired disability?
- Is the disability static or deteriorating?
- Is the disability observable by other people?

Effect of condition on sexuality
- Does the disability effect sexual function or sexuality?
- Does the disability impair cognitive or intellectual ability?
- Are there associated iatrogenic factors?
- Is fertility the principal concern?

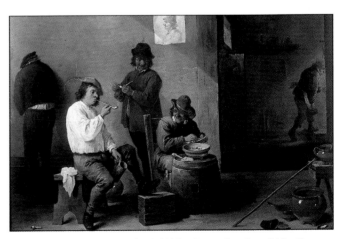

Patients with an impairment that is hidden from others but which affects continence or sexual function often find the situation unbearable (Detail from *Boors Carousing* (1644) by David Teniers the Younger)

Men with cardiac difficulties such as angina often present with sexual problems because they are worried about bringing on an attack if they attempt lovemaking; Women with joint difficulties (such as rheumatoid arthritis and osteoporosis) may find sexual positioning painful and so avoid activity.

Deteriorating conditions
In most cases of trauma patients experience a loss that does not deteriorate, such as spinal cord injury or amputation. However, some conditions like multiple sclerosis do deteriorate (in either a stepwise or gradual manner), which requires mental adjustment to the initial diagnosis and to its reappraisal as the condition worsens. Sexual dysfunction may occur in multiple sclerosis initially as a direct result of demyelination of the nerve and may also be the result of indirect effects as the condition deteriorates. There may be problems with other organ systems as well as fatigue, anxiety, depression, and, indeed, altered desire of the patient's partner. Disability services and general practitioners must address the sexual needs of not only the patients but also their partners at times of need.

Mental impairment
Some conditions such as Huntington's chorea and traumatic brain injury may alter a patient's ability to think in a reasoned way. Injury to the reticular activating system of the pons and midbrain slows arousal, whereas injury to the frontal lobes may result in promiscuity because of reduced inhibition. Indirect effects of brain injury, such as alteration of endocrine function (for example, post-traumatic hypopituitarism), can also affect sexual drive and arousal.

Those with learning difficulties often have problems developing an understanding of their sexual identity. This may be a direct consequence of their learning impairment or a result of overprotection by families. Parents and carers often feel uncomfortable with a child's developing sexual behaviour, possibly because of fear of exploitation or because of their own lack of understanding or acceptance of the child's sexual needs. The patient's general practitioner is often the person to whom family members first mention their worries or may be the first to raise the issue.

Common sexual difficulties

People may have never had a specific sexual experience (primary impairment) or may have become unable to continue with their sex life (secondary impairment). Primary functional impairments—such as a man's inability to get an erection or to ejaculate or a woman's pain, inability to allow penetration, or anorgasmia—are more common among patients with congenital disabilities or those of early onset and are often hard to resolve. Men are more likely to present than women, possibly reflecting cultural perceptions of the importance of sexual performance and, now, the greater range of treatment options available.

Sexual function and arousal in men and women occur in response to reflexogenic genital stimulation or psychogenic desire in those with intact sexual drive mechanisms. Those with brain or spinal cord injury, or whose injury or disease process affects the spinal cord, experience partial or complete loss of sexual functions. They require comprehensive assessment of the level and degree of damage to the brain and nerve cord and the damage to upper and lower motor neurones (by testing the bulbocavernosal and anal wink reflexes; see earlier article by Dean). In neurological terms male erection is similar to the female vasocongestive response and lubrication, and male ejaculation is similar to female contraction of the pelvic floor, perineum, and anal sphincter.

Assessing sexual problems in disabled patients. Do I refer for sexual support?

Mainly psychological cause of problem	Mainly organic cause of problem
• Acute onset	• Generally slower onset
• General relationship with partner (excluding sexual problem) is poor (refer to Relate for appropriate counselling)	• Good, reasonably harmonious relationship with partner
• Symptoms not consistent in all situations	• Symptoms consistent in all situations and with all people
• Major life events (births; deaths; potential or actual change in relationship, health, job) often present	• Major life events rarely present
• Coexisting problem with mental or physical health rarely present	• Coexisting problem with mental or physical health common
• Men with erectile dysfunction have nocturnal or early morning erections	• No nocturnal or early morning erections in men with erectile dysfunction
• Can respond to self stimulation	• No response to self stimulation
• Commonly aged <50 years	• Commonly aged >50 years
• Genitalia (including prostate) and secondary sexual characteristics seem normal	• Genitalia and secondary sexual characteristics show abnormal structure or development
• Normal results from investigations*	• Abnormal results from investigations*
• Refer to psychosexual services for further help	• Refer to suitable specialist for abnormal genitalia and coexisting health problems

*Full blood count; urea and electrolytes; urine analysis; liver function; thyroxin, glucose, and sex hormone concentrations
Adapted from Sefton psychosexual advisory network

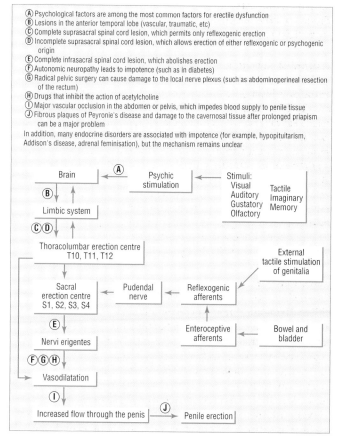

Causes of erectile dysfunction

Effects of drugs

Many disabled people take drugs to control conditions associated with their disability or for pre-existing conditions. Drugs prescribed for medical conditions account for about 25% of cases of erectile dysfunction, and 10% of commonly prescribed drugs produce erectile dysfunction. Overuse of other addictive drugs such as alcohol, tobacco, and cannabis can also disrupt sexual functioning.

Erectile dysfunction

Loss of erectile function is the commonest sexual problem among disabled patients. Even in cases of a clear physical cause, psychological factors are often also important. Physical loss of erection is most often treated by injection of drugs directly into the penis or, recently, with the oral drug sildenafil (Viagra), which has been shown to enhance erectile ability in 70–90% of patients. Vacuum devices can be used by men who do not want to inject themselves, and there are topical preparations, but these are used less often because of their relative lack of success. Patients with erectile dysfunction of primarily psychological origin may benefit from a wide range of specialist psychological therapies, which usually include their partner.

Difficulties with ejaculation

Ejaculatory dysfunction among disabled people is most common in men with spinal cord injury, multiple sclerosis, spina bifida, and transverse myelitis. Ejaculation involves closure of the bladder neck (through sympathetic stimulation) and relaxation of the external sphincter.

Patients with spinal damage often experience retrograde ejaculation into the bladder because of sympathetic damage, and various procedures have been used to induce an ejaculate. In men with an upper motor neurone lesion but with an intact sacral cord, vibratory stimulation is often used. After training, vibratory stimulation of the penis can be attempted at home. Once the frequency and amplitude of the vibration has been selected, the vibrator is applied to the penis to stimulate the pudendal nerve.

If this is unsuccessful patients with lower motor neurone injuries can be helped by electroejaculation. This involves the insertion of a stimulatory probe into the rectum to stimulate the midsacral roots directly, but it requires hospital attendance because of the complexity of the procedure and the potential side effects of pain and autonomic dysreflexia.

Fertility problems

For men with neurological impairment, obtaining semen with a reasonable sperm count and motility is a problem. The same difficulty occurs with many other injuries and as a side effects of drugs used to treat various conditions.

Women with traumatic brain injury, epilepsy, multiple sclerosis, and diabetes retain an anatomically reproductive system, but the physiological effects of their condition may alter ovulation or hormone secretion. The lower pregnancy rates reported in disabled women are probably the result of conception being avoided because of concerns over their ability to raise a family as well as manage their impairment. Those with congenital disorders known to affect fertility and childbirth should be given the opportunity to discuss any anxieties with a genetic counsellor.

Assisted conception

Technology exists to obtain ejaculate from most men, but the problem of semen quality, particular sperm motility, remains. The reason for this is unclear, although scrotal hyperthermia, long term use of certain drugs, prolonged sitting in a

---

Drugs that can cause erectile dysfunction*

Antipsychotics, anxiolytics, hypnotics
- Phenothiazines—such as chlorpromazine
- Butyrophenones—such as haloperidol
- Benzodiazepines

Anticholinergics
- Atropine
- Diphenhydramine—such as in over the counter cold remedies and sleeping pills

Hormones
- Corticosteroids
- Oestrogens
- Anabolic steroids (high dose)

Antiandrogens

Antidepressants
- Tricyclics—such as amitriptyline, imipramine, dothiepin
- Monoamine oxidase inhibitors— such as phenelzine
- selective serotonin reuptake inhibitors—may cause ejaculatory problems

Antihypertensives
- Diuretics—such as thiazides, spironolactone
- Vasodilators
- Central sympatholytics—such as methyldopa, clonidine, reserpine
- Ganglion blockers—such as guanethidine, bethanidine
- β blockers—such as propanolol, metoprolol, atenolol
- ACE inhibitors—such as enalapril
- Calcium channel blockers—such as nifedipine

Dopamine antagonists
- Metoclopramide

H_2 antagonists
- Cimetidine

Psychotropic drugs
- Alcohol
- Cannabis
- Amphetamines
- Barbiturates
- Opioids
- Tobacco smoking

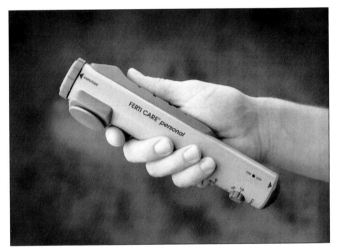

Ferticare personal vibrator—developed to help men with spinal cord injuries to ejaculate and is effective in 80% of cases

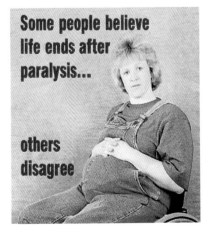

Some people believe life ends after paralysis... others disagree

Options exist for improving sexual function and fertility for those with a wide range of disabling conditions

wheelchair, and repeated urinary tract infections have all been suggested.

At the simplest level, couples can be taught how to obtain semen with a vibrator at home and introduce it into the vagina with a standard syringe. If sperm motility is low (<35%) in vitro fertilisation can be useful. The process is also helpful for some men with spinal cord injury.

The recently developed techniques of microassisted fertilisation require only small numbers of motile sperm. Intracytoplasmic sperm injection, in which semen is inserted directly into the egg cytoplasm, is more suited for those with low sperm counts. Research indicates fertilisation rates as high as 70% and childbirth rates as high as those with in vitro fertilisation. Studies are currently assessing the effectiveness of using a small specimen of semen taken directly from the epididymis for in vitro fertilisation or intracytoplasmic sperm injection.

Even in conditions of severe disability, such as tetraplegia, close monitoring by a team of specialists including the spinal injury team and urological and gynaecological services should ensure maximum likelihood of conception and pregnancy. Options exist for improving sexual function and fertility for those with a wide range of disabling conditions. Such people do not wish for preferential treatment, but they do deserve equal opportunity of access to a fulfilling sex life.

Further help

Your local spinal injury centre should be able to advise on the availability of services for disabled people in the area

Spinal injury centres are at

- Hexham General Hospital, Hexham NE46 1QJ (Tel 01434 606161)
- Musgrave Park Hospital, Belfast BT9 7JB (Tel 028 9066 9501)
- Northern General Hospital, Sheffield S5 7AU (Tel 0114 2434343)
- Our Lady of Lourdes Hospital, Dun Laoghaire, Dublin, Republic of Ireland (Tel 00 353 528 5477)
- Pinderfields General Hospital, Wakefield WF1 4EE (Tel 01924 201688)
- Robert Jones and Agnes Hunt Orthopaedic Hospital, Oswestry ST10 7AG (Tel 01691 404000)
- Rookwood Hospital, Cardiff CF5 2YN (Tel 029 2056 6281)
- Royal National Orthopaedic Hospital, Stanmore HA7 4LP (Tel 0181 954 2300)
- Salisbury District General Hospital, Salisbury SP2 8BJ (Tel 01722 336262)
- Southern General Hospital, Glasgow G51 4TF (Tel 0141 2012555)
- Southport District General Hospital, Southport PR8 6PN (Tel 01704 547471)
- Stoke Mandeville Hospital, Aylesbury HP21 8AL (Tel 01296 315000)

Other support:

- Spinal Injury Association, 76 St James Lane, London N10 3DF (Tel 0181 444 2121)
- Multiple Sclerosis Society, 25 Effie Road, London SW6 1EE (Tel 0171 610 7171)
- SPOD (Association to aid the sexual and personal relationships of people with disability), 288 Camden Road, London N7 0BJ (Tel 0171 607 8851)
- British Diabetic Assocaition, 10 Queen Anne Street, London W1M 0BD (Tel 0171 323 1531)
- The Impotence Association, PO Box 10296, London SW17 7ZN (Tel 0181 767 7791)

Autonomic dysreflexia and hyperreflexia

Untreated, the condition is life threatening and can result in convulsions, cerebral haemorrhage, and death

- Occurs in spinal cord lesions above T6
- Due to increased autonomic activity after stimulus (such as distended bowel or bladder)
- Signal from the receptor travels up the spinal column until blocked at the level of the lesion
- Local vasoconstriction responses are activated, and the person experiences intense headache due to rapid rise in blood pressure
- Parasympathetic response to try to stabilise blood pressure cannot travel down the spinal cord past the level of the lesion, and so the blood pressure continues to rise

Management

- At first sign of symptoms (flushing, serious sweating above lesion level, nasal congestion, extreme headache) take immediate action to determine the cause and remove the stimulus
- Sublingual nifedipine can be used to lower the blood pressure

The posters for the Spinal Injuries Association were reproduced with permission of the SIA, and the photographs were by Jim Kelly. The painting by Teniers is reproduced with permission of the Bridgeman Art Library Wallace Collection.

Jane Read

Sexuality and infertility

Infertility may interact with a couple's or individual's sexuality and sexual expression in two main ways. Sexual problems may be caused or exacerbated by the diagnosis, investigation, and management of infertility (or subfertility), or they may be a contributory factor in childlessness. Any examination of a couple's difficulty in conceiving must include overt and clear questioning about their sexual activity.

Responses to infertility

In response to being unable to conceive, many people feel emotions such as anger, panic, despair, and grief, and these may have several effects on sexual activity. The stress of infertility and its treatment may be a cause of sexual difficulties for both the prospective father and mother.

Intercourse may be avoided, with patterns of behaviour established, so that one or other partner is not reminded of the fertility problem. Postcoital tests or having to provide semen samples may result in a man feeling under pressure to perform, adversely affecting his erectile or ejaculatory ability. For some men, one or two failures during intercourse begins a vicious circle of fear of failure, with anxiety leading to further failures. Partners may also develop arousal difficulties because of anxiety or distress. Some individuals feel that their partner seems to want them only when there is a chance of conception, and sexual activity can then become a battleground for issues of power and control.

These stresses all conspire to alienate the couple from the recreational aspects of sexual expression and focus them, sometimes obsessively, on the procreative aspect of sexual intercourse.

Sexual problems that result in infertility

Childlessness may be the result of an existing sexual dysfunction. One study of infertile couples found that 5% had a history of sexual problems.

To avoid wasting time and resources, it is important that patients are given the opportunity to discuss their previous pattern of sexual functioning, to see if it has changed in the light of their fertility problems. It seems inexcusable that people can undergo months or years of invasive and expensive treatment when simple, clear questions about their sexual lives may elicit information that could spare them the ordeal. Infertility examinations should therefore include an evaluation of couples' sexual behaviour, with special reference to frequency and timing of coitus.

Two further categories of sexual dysfunction need to be borne in mind. The first is retrograde ejaculation, in which, at orgasm, the ejaculate is expelled back into the bladder rather than externally. This can be checked fairly simply by examining a postejaculatory urine sample for the presence of sperm. Men with this condition experience "dry" orgasm, feeling the sensation of muscular action and orgasm but not producing an ejaculate. This is a fairly common presentation in fertility units and can be managed medically by centrifuging the urine to collect the sperm.

The second point to consider is whether the sperm are being introduced into the vagina. This can mean talking in

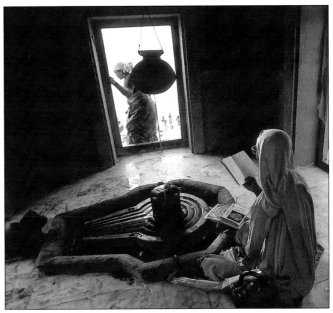

Fertility has always been vitally important in human society, and its absence can lead to anger, panic, despair, and grief, which may have several effects on sexual activity. (Photograph shows prayers being read before a lingam, the phallic symbol of Shiva, Hindu god of fertility)

Useful questions to elicit information*

- How have your fertility problems affected your relationship, including your sexual relationship?
- Has anything changed in your sexual relationship since you have been trying to conceive?
- How would you describe your sexual activity?
- How often do you have penetrative (that is, penis in vagina) sex?

*Taken from Read J. *Counselling for fertility problems.* London: Sage, 1995:104

Sexual problems commonly associated with infertility

Male problems
- Loss of desire, with a consequent decrease in sexual activity
- Erectile problems
- Premature ejaculation—little or no control over ejaculatory response, and ejaculation may occur before vaginal entry achieved
- Retarded ejaculation—difficulty ejaculating intravaginally, or at all

Female problems
- Loss of desire
- Vaginismus
- Dyspareunia
- Anorgasmia

very clear terms to the couple about the nature of their sexual activity. Some couples engage in anal intercourse, in umbilical sex, or in manual stimulation alone and somewhat naively consider that their sexual behaviour is normal and should be resulting in pregnancy.

Sexual difficulties in pregnancy

Pregnancy is a transition from one physical state to another. In the case of a first pregnancy it is a transition from one state of being to another—from being a couple to being a family, from being a person in relationship with another to motherhood or fatherhood. As with any transition, there is a sense of loss as well as excitement at entering another phase of life's experience.

It is important to remember that pregnancy is not always met with joy and that, even if a baby is planned and wanted, there may be some ambivalence: "Neither pregnancy nor its absence is inherently desirable. The occurrence of a pregnancy can be met with joy or despair, and its absence can be a cause of relief or anguish. Whether these states are wanted, the conscious or unconscious meanings attached to pregnancy and infertility, the responses of others, the perceived implications of these states and expectations for the future are all critical factors in determining an individual's response."[1]

Included in this response will be myths about pregnancy, taboos about sexual activity during pregnancy, fears about the baby and delivery, changes in the relationship with the partner, and beliefs about the roles of motherhood and fatherhood. The woman's changing body shape may cause distress and a sense of unattractiveness.

This ambivalence may become manifest in sexual difficulties that are essentially psychological in origin, as an emotional response to the changed or changing state, or they may be a direct physical response to the pregnancy. One, of course, does not exclude the other, and a mixed aetiology is common.[2] There may be a combination of sexual problems, and they may also occur in the period after delivery. A careful history should be taken to ascertain what is causing any difficulties.

Psychological factors

In cases when pregnancy is the result of infertility treatment or when there is a history of repeated miscarriages, fetal handicap, or neonatal death there may be high levels of anxiety, with repeated requests for reassurance or perhaps demands for scans or examinations. Apart from general anxiety, there may be specific concerns about body image, delivery, motherhood, changes to the couple's relationship, miscarriage, lack of self esteem, sexual guilt, and tiredness.

Myths about intercourse during pregnancy include the fear it may cause miscarriage, premature labour, or fetal damage. Savage and Reader confirmed that there is no significant increase in fetal problems in women who continue to be sexually active throughout pregnancy.[3] They noted that 27% of these women had uterine contractions after orgasm that were sometimes painful. Those who experienced painful contractions were less likely to have sexual intercourse often or at all.

There are, however, obvious indications for abstaining from intercourse during pregnancy,[4] which include
- Vaginal bleeding
- Placenta praevia
- Premature dilatation of the cervix
- Rupture of the membranes
- History of premature delivery
- Multiple pregnancy.

Physical factors associated with pregnancy that can reduce sexual activity*
- Tiredness
- Backache
- Dyspareunia
  Pelvic vasocongestion
  Vaginal congestion with reduced lubrication
  Subluxation of pubic symphysis and sacroiliac joints
  Retroverted uterus, particularly in first weeks of pregnancy
  Weight of partner on uterus during intercourse in late pregnancy
  Deep engagement of fetal head
  Candida and trichomonas infections
- Haemorrhoids
- Urinary tract infections
- Stress incontinence
- Vulval varicose veins

*Data from Reamy KJ, White SE. Dyspareunia in pregnancy. *J Psychosom Obstet Gynaecol* 1985;4:263

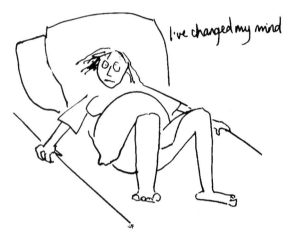

Pregnancy is not always met with joy, and even if a baby is planned and wanted there may be some ambivalence

---

Points to consider when taking a history
- Assessment of relationship, sexually and otherwise, and the support network
- Whether the pregnancy was planned
- Previous pregnancies and outcomes (such as miscarriage, termination)
- Previous deliveries—type and presence of trauma
- Current children's health
- Contraception—past and current use and plans for the future

---

Sexual problems during or after pregnancy

Female problems
- Loss of libido associated with tiredness, negative body image, etc
- Anorgasmia associated with lack of arousal or pain
- Vaginismus associated with pain or trauma from delivery

Male problems
- Lack of desire
- Erectile dysfunction associated with fears raised by watching the delivery, causing pain on intercourse, fatherhood
- Premature ejaculation associated with fears raised by watching the delivery, causing pain on intercourse, fatherhood

Sexuality and ageing

Bancroft reported that there has been a widespread tendency to assume that elderly people are too old for sex activity and the sexuality of both men and women declines with advancing years.[5] This decline depends on three main factors: the level of sexual activity throughout a person's lifetime, physical health, and psychological health.

Sexuality throughout life

People who have been sexually active on a frequent basis throughout their life will show a lower rate of decline in activity with advancing years than will those who have been less sexually active. Most elderly people who remain sexually active experience high enjoyment from sex,[6] and, in a summary of studies on sex and ageing, Kaplan concluded that most physically healthy men and women remain sexually active on a regular basis into their ninth decade.[7]

What form this sexual activity takes could include solo and mutual masturbation, oral sex, and penetrative intercourse. It is essential to remember that elderly people may have just as wide a range of interests and preferences as younger people.

Physical health

Any condition or illness can have an impact on sexual function. For example, a woman with severe arthritis may have difficulties with using her hands to pleasure herself or her partner or finding a sexual position that minimises the pain. Careful positioning of pillows may help with the latter problem.

Patients may find it very difficult to raise subjects such as managing incontinence in sexual contact with another person and in solo masturbation, and it requires great sensitivity by the doctor to uncover such concerns. The use of appropriate creams to help with vaginal soreness—such as oestrogen cream (if the woman is not already taking hormone replacement therapy), KY Jelly or Senselle, or an aromatic oil such as sweet almond or peach kernel oil (but not to be used with latex contraceptives, which perish)—may enable a woman (and her partner) to enjoy sexual activity much more fully. Giving patients "permission" to use vibrators to assist with access to genital areas and stimulation is often helpful.

Psychological health

Myths and beliefs about sexual attractiveness and what it is may affect older women and contribute to low self esteem and possibly depression. A woman who has been widowed may find difficulty in finding a new partner because of the higher ratio of women to men in older age groups.

Elderly people may be embarrassed or ashamed of having sexual needs "at their age," and they may feel fear and guilt about indulging in sexual behaviour after having been in a long term relationship, in effect a form of performance anxiety. For women especially, there may also be family expectations of celibacy that may be difficult to counter and other social expectations that elderly people are no longer sexual.

1 Adler N. Foreword. In: Stanton AL, Dunken-Schetter C, eds. *Infertility. Perspectives from stress and coping research.* New York: Plenum Publishing, 1991.
2 Guano-Trujillo B, Higgins P. Sexual intercourse and pregnancy. *Health Care Wom Int* 1987;5:339.
3 Savage W, Reader F. Sexual activity during pregnancy. *Midwife Health Visitor Community Nurse* 1984;20:398.
4 Mills JL, Harlap S, Harley EE. Should coitus late in pregnancy be discouraged? *Lancet* 1981;ii:136.
5 Bancroft J. *Human sexuality and its problems.* 2nd ed. Edinburgh: Churchill Livingstone, 1989:282-5.
6 Brecher EM. *Love, sex and ageing. Consumer's Union report.* Boston, MA: Little, Brown, 1984.
7 Kaplan HS. Injection treatment for older patients. In: Wagner G, Kaplan HS, eds. *The new injection treatment for impotence.* New York: Brunner, Mazel, 1993:142.

Percentage of older men and women who are sexually active and find it enjoyable*

	Age group (years)		
	50-59	60-69	70-79
Sexually active subjects			
All women (n=1844):	93	81	65
Married (n=1245)	95	89	81
Unmarried (n=512)	98	63	50
All men (n=2402):	98	91	79
Married (n=1895)	98	93	81
Unmarried (n=414)	95	85	75
Sex highly enjoyable (sexually active subjects)			
Women	71	65	61
Men	90	86	75

*Data from Brecher (1984)[6]

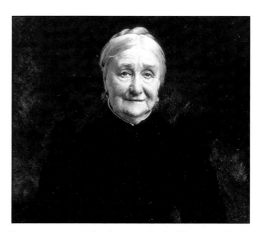

For women especially, there may be family expectations of celibacy and social expectations that elderly people are no longer sexual. (Detail of *Madame Bonnat, the artist's mother* (1893) by Leon Joseph Florentin Bonnat)

Health factors that inhibit sexual activity in elderly people

Physical factors
- Stress incontinence
- Diminishing mobility
- Decreasing muscle tone
- Uterine prolapse
- Skin tone and sensitivity
- Diseases such as diabetes and cardiovascular problems
- Chronic conditions such as arthritis

Psychological health
- Sense of unattractiveness
- Facing mortality; depression, bereavement and grief reactions
- Loss of partner or friends
- Lack of contact with others and loneliness

Further reading
- Read J. *Counselling for fertility problems.* London: Sage, 1995
- Reamy KJ, White SE. Dyspareunia in pregnancy. *J Psychosom Obstet Gynaecol* 1985;4:263

The photograph of a Shiva lingam is reproduced with permission of the Hutchinson Library. The cartoon "I've changed my mind" is reproduced with permission of Jacky Fleming from *Be a Bloody Train Driver.* The painting by Bonnat is reproduced with permission of Lauros-Giraudon and the Bridgeman Art Library.

16 Sexual variations

W P de Silva

"Sexual variations" refer to sexual desires and behaviours outside what is considered to be the normal range, although what is unusual or atypical varies between cultures and from one period to another. Defining normality is extremely difficult (and arbitrary), because the definition involves making a value judgment and therefore labelling how we view other people.

Sexual variations are also referred to as paraphilias, a neutral term for behaviours formerly called deviant. They can be defined as conditions in which a person's sexual gratification is dependent on an unusual sexual experience revolving round particular sex objects.[1] They are much more common in men than women.

History and culture

Sexual variations have existed and been recorded for millennia in different parts of the world. For example, early Buddhist texts contain numerous references to sexually variant behaviours among monastic communities over 2000 years ago. These behaviours included sexual activity with animals and sexual interest in corpses.

In the clinical literature sexual variations had begun to be extensively discussed by the second half of the 19th century. The classic example is Richard von Krafft-Ebing's *Psychopathia Sexualis*, first published in 1887. In this book the author, a neuropsychiatrist, details, among others, fetishism, flagellation, sadism, necrophilia, sadistic acts with animals, masochism, exhibitionism, bondage, paedophilia, bestiality, and incest.

Major sexual variations

Exhibitionism is among the most common of the sexual variations. The usual image is of a middle aged man in a dirty raincoat "flashing." Typically, however, exhibitionists are postpubescent males up to the age of 40 who obtain high levels of sexual pleasure and excitement from exposing their genitals to females, usually strangers, and who may masturbate at the same time.

Paedophilia involves intense sexual urges and sexual activity with prepubescent children. Two thirds of molested children are girls, usually between the ages of 8 and 11. To meet the diagnostic criteria, a paedophile must be at least 16 years old and at least five years older than the victim. Most paedophiles are men, but there are cases of women having repeated sexual contact with children. In 90% of cases the molester is known to the child, and 15% (possibly more) are relatives. Most paedophiles are heterosexual and are often married with their own children, although they commonly have marital or sexual difficulties or problems with alcohol misuse. Eighty per cent have a history of childhood sexual abuse.

Fetishism involves recurrent sexual urges or behaviours concerning the use of inanimate objects such as leather and rubber garments, women's underwear, stockings, and shoes and boots.

Transvestism refers to recurrent, intense sexually arousing fantasies, urges, and behaviours involving cross dressing. A transvestite is a heterosexual male who derives sexual satisfaction by wearing female clothing. Many are married and seem very masculine. They should not be mistaken for female impersonators on the stage (such as "Dame Edna Everage") or male homosexuals who cross dress ("go in drag"), who are

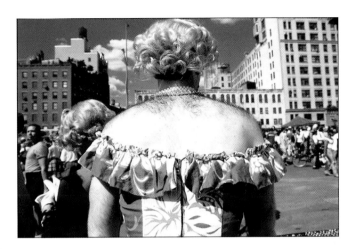

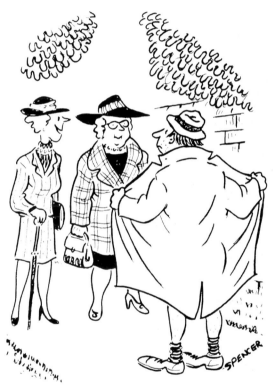

" You don't often see a real silk lining, these days . . ."

A case example of fetishism from Krafft-Ebing (1887)

Z began to masturbate at the age of 12. From that time he could not see a woman's handkerchief without having orgasm and ejaculation. He was irresistibly compelled to possess himself of it. At that time he was a choir boy and used the handkerchiefs to masturbate within the bell tower close to the choir. But he chose only such handkerchiefs as had black and white borders or violet stripes running through them. At age 15, he had coitus. Later on he married. As a rule, he was potent only when he wound such a handkerchief around his penis. Often he preferred coitus between the thighs of a woman where he had placed a handkerchief. Whenever he espied a handkerchief, he did not rest until he was in possession of it. He always had a number of them in his pockets and around his penis

---

not sexually aroused or dependent on their cross dressing for sexual excitement.

Transsexualism is not, strictly speaking, a paraphilia but rather an issue of gender role. Transsexuals have an intense desire to become a member of the opposite sex, feeling that they are trapped in the "wrong body." Many therefore ask for surgical intervention for a sex change. Transsexualism is found equally in males and females, and they should not be confused with transvestites, who cross dress for sexual arousal but who do not want anatomical change.

Hypoxyphilia is an increasingly commonly reported variation that involves attempts to enhance the pleasure of orgasm by a reduction of oxygen intake—for example, by placing a tight noose around one's neck. Such behaviour has lead to fatalities.

Other sexual variations include gaining sexual pleasure from inflicting pain (sadism) or from suffering pain or humiliation (masochism), sexual desire for corpses (necrophilia) or for animals (zoophilia or bestiality), arousal from contact with urine (urophilia) and faeces (coprophilia), and excitement from rubbing the genitals against a clothed person in a confined space such as the Underground (frotteurism).

Combinations—It is not unusual for an individual to have more than one sexual variation. The commonest combination is fetishism, transvestism, sadism, and masochism.

Clinical presentations

Sexual variations seen in clinical settings are only a proportion of the cases where such problems exist. There are, broadly speaking, four classes of clinical referral.
• Those sent for clinical intervention by the law enforcing authorities. These are sex offenders who are asked to have treatment to help them overcome their problem behaviour.
• Those who seek help for their sexual variations because they are distressed by them. These include people who worry that they might commit illegal or embarrassing acts. Many are distressed by acts they see as "unnatural" or are afraid that they may endanger their life or their career.
• Those who seek help because their partners are distressed by the sexual variation. They are themselves distressed because of their partner's distress. These are people with stable or long term relationships.
• Those who present with frank sexual dysfunction. They report erectile difficulties or other dysfunctions, which are usually secondary to strong variant desires and reliance on these for arousal. For example, a man may find that he is unable to sustain an erection for sexual intercourse with his partner unless he has contact with, say, a leather garment.

Assessment

Clinical assessment in these cases needs to be comprehensive, with information elicited about a number of aspects. These include variant arousal and sexual fantasies, anxiety about problems with conventional sexual stimuli such as consenting adult partners, anxiety or difficulties with social interaction with adults of the same age group who are potential sexual partners, or whether the person has a problem with his or her gender.

Treatment

The aims of treatment must be carefully considered, and the therapist and the client need to arrive at an agreed goal. Until about 20 years ago, most patients were treated with one aim only—to eliminate their variant sexual arousal. The main technique used was electrical aversion therapy. This often suppressed the problem behaviour but did not eliminate it and its use is now uncommon.

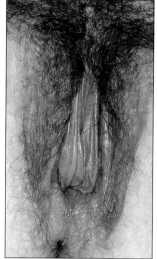
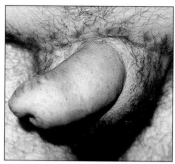

Results of surgery for change of sex. Left: final appearance of male to female change. Right: female to male change, still bruised at one week after operation

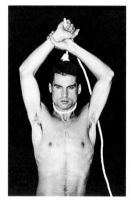

Hypoxyphilia is an increasingly common attempt to enhance orgasm by reducing oxygen intake

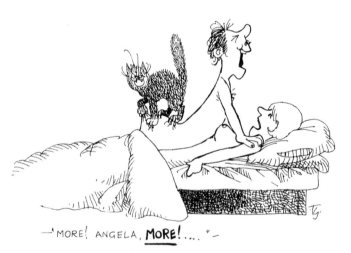

—"MORE! ANGELA, MORE!...."—

People may seek help for their sexual variations because their partners are distressed by the variation

> **Treatment of sexual variations is difficult. After careful assessment, treatment goals must be established, and, to achieve these, a comprehensive therapeutic package is usually needed. Focusing on the variant arousal is only one aspect of treatment, and therapy that takes this as the sole focus is rarely successful**

If the goal of treatment is to eliminate the sexual variation, it must be recognised that success may be limited. Control may be achieved, but this needs to be supplemented with gains in other, more acceptable, sexual behaviours. In practice, this means that any treatment programme that includes an attempt to get rid of the variation must also include enhancement of other outlets. Other sexual anxieties or skills deficits need to be addressed.

Incorporation

An alternative to elimination is to incorporate the variation in a controlled way into the person's sexual repertoire. This is especially so in the case of people whose partners are distressed by the dominant role of the variation in their sexual behaviour. Obviously, this is not possible if the variation is unacceptable, such as paedophilia. It is also important that the variation is something the partner can tolerate in a limited way.

In practice, the therapist will use a multifaceted therapy programme. One aspect of such a programme is conventional sex therapy, aimed at enhancing the sexual relationship. In further joint work, the couple are helped to systematically reduce the role of the variation in their sexual relationship. For example, a man with a rubber or leather fetish may be asked to wear only a leather arm band during sex. Similarly, temporal control may be introduced, using a timetable approach. The couple agree, for example, to use the fetish object in their sexual relations on certain days of the week only.

Group therapy

Some clinics operate group therapy programmes. These are most commonly used for sex offenders. The programmes involve group processes and group learning.

Chemical treatment

For those with serious difficulties, chemical treatment is sometimes considered. Reduction of the sex drive through drugs will, of course, reduce the problem behaviour, but its effectiveness is not selective: that is, the drive is dampened down in toto, not just the desire for the variant behaviour. The drugs commonly used are medroxyprogesterone acetate and cyproterone acetate.

Orgasmic reconditioning

This approach has been used since the 1970s, and its main feature is the reinforcement of conventional arousal and desires. Typically, the patient is asked to masturbate with his variant fantasy and then, when orgasm is imminent (the point of no return), to switch to a fantasy of a conventional sexual stimulus or behaviour. The ensuing orgasm then powerfully reinforces the conventional desire. In succeeding sessions (which the client carries out in privacy) the point when the switching is made is brought forward so that, eventually, the entire sequence takes place to conventional fantasies.

Aversion therapy

A related procedure to electrical aversion is covert sensitisation. Here, the aversion is covert and imagined. The person is asked to fantasise a sequence of events involving his or her variant behaviour and, at a crucial point of the sequence, to imagine a powerful aversive scene. For example, a paedophiliac might be asked to imagine the appearance of a police officer at the point of his approaching a child in his sequence of images. The aversive scenes are agreed in advance, and typically more than one aversive consequence is used.

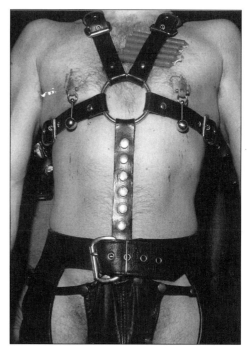

In couple therapy a man with a leather fetish may be encouraged to reduce his use of the fetish to a level more acceptable to his partner

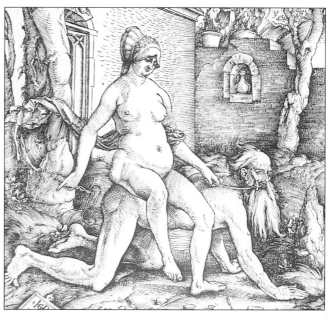

With orgasmic reconditioning, a man is asked to change his variant fantasy to one of conventional sexual behaviour while masturbating. (Detail of *Phyllis Riding Aristotle* (1513) by Hans Baldung Grien)

1 Masters WH, Johnson VE, Kolodny RC. *Human sexuality.* 5th ed. New York: Harper Collins, 1995.

The photographs of a transvestite, by Anne Maniglier, and a man wearing leather gear, by Gordon Rainsford, are reproduced with permission of Gaze International. The cartoon "You don't often see a real silk lining. . ." is reproduced with permission of Punch Publications. The cartoon "More, Angela, more" is reproduced with permission of Tony Goffe.

17 Sex aids

Christopher Headon, Margot Huish

Sex aids vary from mechanical aids for production of an orgasm, such as vibrators, to visual aids such as pornographic material and specialist clothing for variational sex. Aids to produce and maintain an erection are dealt with in other chapters, as are aids for production of ejaculate in men with spinal injuries. This section details sex aids for pleasure and stimulation, and the medical problems that they can cause.

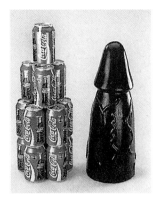

Standard mechanical aids

Vibrators are used for clitoral, vaginal, penile, and anal stimulation. They can be battery operated or mains driven, in various materials, and phallic in shape or in various other shapes for stimulation externally or internally. "Love eggs" can be inserted into the vagina or rectum, and the vibration triggered by remote control. Wires must be safely housed within the device, as they could traumatise tissue or cause an electric shock if they were pulled loose. Vibrators made to plug into car cigarette lighters could prove hazardous if used while driving.

Dildos can be used for clitoral, vaginal, and anal stimulation. These are non-vibrating phallic shaped devices manufactured from latex, very occasionally inflatable, that are hand held or strapped on to a harness. Clearly, these are visually as well as physically exciting. Dangers include the tearing of vaginal and anal linings through overenthusiastic use, possibly under the influence of "poppers," which seem to reduce the perception of pain (see below). There is also the risk of infection if dildos are shared between partners. Accident and emergency departments have encountered patients who have used coat hangers, light bulbs, and bottles as dildos, and who were too embarrassed to visit their general practitioner.

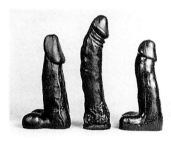

The dangers of using dildos include the tearing of vaginal or anal linings through overenthusiastic use

Inflatable dolls—A life size male or female plastic companion can be used for sex and never refuses any request.

Ticklers are attached to a condom or erect penis to enhance clitoral and vaginal stimulation.

Aids in sadomasochistic sex

While "rough" or sadomasochistic sex is a separate category, there are obviously crossovers into more regular forms of sexual activity.

Mechanical aids

Butt plugs are devices to be inserted into the anus to stretch it and give a sense of anal fullness. They are generally rubber, sometimes stainless steel or leather, and are usually conical but sometimes round in shape. Occasionally, they are attached to a harness or rubber pants and are sometimes used in preparation for inserting a larger dildo or a fist.

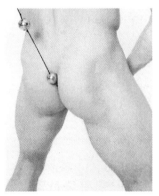

"Love balls" can also be inserted into the anus

Love Balls connected by a cord and in a variety of sizes, can also be inserted in the anus.

Duck billed specula—These gynaecological instruments are effectively reverse pliers and can be used for anal enlargement. They may be painful and dangerous in inexpert hands.

Nipple clamps are for attaching to the nipple to produce painful or pleasurable "highs" through the release of endorphins. They usually come with a spring or screw bar and are mainly padded with rubber; rarely, they are tubing clamps that are screwed down on the nipple. A clothes peg is an example of a simple nipple clamp.

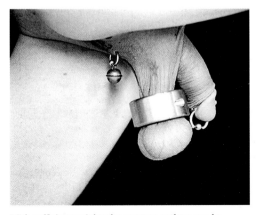

With sufficient weight, the scrotum and vas can be stretched to great lengths

Ball toys—A wide range of toys for playing with testicles are available, including straps, stretchers, and weights. With sufficient weights, the scrotum and vasa can be stretched to great lengths.

Piercing of genitals, nipples, and other body parts

Thin needles can be inserted into the penis or labia for physical and visual stimulation, but more usual is the insertion of body jewellery such as rings, which can be pulled or have a weight attached to them. Piercings are becoming fashionable outside the sadomasochistic community, especially rings or studs through the nose, lips, ears, eyebrows, tongue, and umbilicus.

Regular cleaning of the piercing with chlorhexidine gluconate 4% (Savlon) solution helps to prevent infection, but if it does get infected, usually with *Staphylococcus aureus*, the patient should not be advised to remove it as the hole will close over and fibrose. Tea tree oil can be used first, but if this is not effective a five day course of antibiotic such as flucloxacillin should be given and the cleaning continued at least twice a day. Unfortunately, patients are often too embarrassed to show a ring or bar bell in an unusual place to their general practitioner.

Some writers link the psychology of piercing with the desire to find roots in the primitive and to have a sense of belonging to a special tribe, and the history of body piercing or adornment in African and Polynesian tribes is long and well respected.

Bondage

Restraints are used for exercising regulation and control. Many devices and practices fall into this category, and problems can arise with any of them. Fettering suggests the historic background of the jail, the prisoner being submissive and in abject humility. Although restraints used in bondage and discipline sessions are sometimes used interchangeably in sadomasochistic sex, a useful distinction in motivation can be made. Generally, bondage is involved in practices with domination, role playing, and humiliation but includes little or no pain, unlike flagellation.

Flagellation and beating

Devotees of flagellation inflict beatings for sexually stimulating torture and punishment. Practices include beating the feet (a form of punishment called "bastinado") spanking, caning, birching, and belting. There is an accompanying range of sexual furniture, such as a wooden horse, crosses, stocks, and suspending equipment. Specific clothing made of tight rubber may also be used to heighten erotic sensation.

Other sadomasochistic games

Enemas and forced feeding through orogastric or nasogastric tubes may be used for control and heightened awareness. Enthusiastic overuse has obvious dangers.

Abrasion—Some men find benefit in stimulating the surface of the body with abrasive materials, and this may become a necessary part of sexual stimulation for orgasm to occur.

Breath control games (asphyxiaphilia) involve restriction of the oxygen supply to the brain. This can be simple (a plastic bag over the head) or more complex (gas masks with a blocked air supply). Death is not uncommon. Autoerotic asphyxiation is called "solo play" and can be the most dangerous sex game employed. There may be sensual pleasure from the constriction itself as well as the excitement of danger. There have been some well publicised deaths from this in the past few years. After vasovagal attacks, fits are the next most common medical emergency, and it has been suggested that, if regularly induced, they can cause cumulative brain damage.

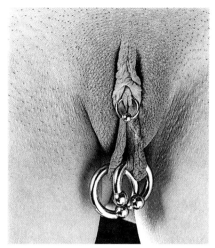

More usual is the insertion of body jewellery such as rings in the penis or labia, which can be pulled or have weights attached

---

Toys used in sadomasochistic sex

Gags represent the surrender of the faculty of speech and demonstrate deep submission. They are made in a wide range of shapes. Because of dangers of suffocation, it is important that recreational drugs are not used in conjunction with them

Hoods and helmets in leather or rubber have important psychological effects: by removing a person's ability to see, hear, taste, or smell, they achieve the sensation of the head being separated from the body

Blindfolds are used to block vision to allow for greater vulnerability and concentration and to encourage a sense of the unexpected

Hospital restraints such as strait jackets, bed or table restraints, and the use of splints and bandages

Sleep sacks and body bags where the body is held within a dark and restrictive place. The body can be "mummified" through the use of cling film and "gaffa" tape (strong woven adhesive tape).

Bondage gear includes handcuffs, ankle restraints, ropes, and chains. Genital bondage for men includes "cock rings," cages, sheaths, and chastity belts (also for women)

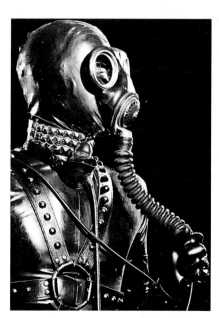

Breath control games involve restriction of the oxygen supply to the brain. Death is not uncommon

Medical aspects of sadomasochistic sex

It is crucial for a medical practitioner to be sensitive to the meanings that the various aspects of sadomasochistic play have for a patient. Bruises found on routine examination might cause a doctor anxiety but not worry the patient, who has willingly received them. The practices of "yellow" sex (playing with urine, urolagnia) and "brown" sex (playing with faeces) might arouse concern about the risk of infection, but the patient is expressing deep psychic and relational needs.

In ethical terms, sadomasochistic play should be consensual, safe, and sane—you can hurt but not harm. The last point ties in with "the spanner case."

Drugs used in sexual activity

The enjoyment of all the senses and the capacity of the human imagination lie at the basis of sexual stimulation, and some people will find simple massage with aromatic oils stimulating while others will swear by special aphrodisiac foods such as oysters and shellfish. The use of drugs during sex is a large subject, but it is useful to focus on examples of clinical interest.

Lignocaine is sold in sex shops as a spray to delay ejaculation. Its anaesthetic action, however, may well dull sensation in the partner who receives the penis.

Ecstasy (methylene dioxymeth amphetamine)—Users report that their enjoyment of sex is heightened through an increase of loving feelings and that orgasm is delayed. A danger is that lowered inhibitions may lead to anal sex without using condoms and therefore possible HIV infection. Other amphetamines also produce euphoria, improve sexual functioning, and delay ejaculation.

Vasodilators (such as butyl nitrate, amyl nitrate, glyceryl trinitrate, and isosorbide dinitrate) in some of their forms are sold as "poppers" in small bottles (sometimes ampoules) from which vapour is inhaled. They work by liberation of nitrous oxide, a smooth muscle relaxant. There is a sensation of "rush" followed by a short lived euphoria, with intensification of current positive emotions. They are often used by gay men as muscle relaxation allows for easier anal intercourse and enhances orgasm. It is suspected, but with no firm evidence, that these drugs depress the immune system.

Cocaine has been described as increasing sexual desire but making erection and ejaculation more difficult. Powdered on to the glans or the clitoris, it acts as a local anaesthetic, delaying orgasm and prolonging intercourse. Placed within the anus, it has a similar anaesthetic effect, but the danger is that the receiver of a fist may be unaware of the pain and damage caused by too vigorous thrusting.

Cannabis is reported to enhance sexual feelings and the sense of touch, while increasing relaxation and pleasure. There seems to be a placebo effect, with those who expect enhancement getting it, while those who have no such expectations do not.

Pornography

Books, magazines, films, videos, music, and advertisements can all be aids to sexual excitement. They can make people feel happy, content in themselves, relaxed, focused, and stimulated whether they are alone or with a partner, but they can have many different meanings for those who use them. For example, a man collecting pornography may be unconsciously attacking his partner, whom he sees as not giving him everything that the models in the magazines would. There is no established evidence that pornography makes people act out sociopathologically, such as causing men to commit rape.

"The spanner case"

The police discovered a home made video in which explicit gay sadomasochism was shown, performed by sadomasochistic participants. After an investigation called "Operation Spanner" these participants were charged with "conspiracy to corrupt public morals" and then, more seriously, with Offences Against the Person Act. All the activities were carried out in private and were consensual. Nevertheless, Judge Rant ruled that consent was no defence to a charge of assault. Two appeals and, finally, the European Court of Human Rights upheld the verdict (*Times* 20 February 1997, p 34)

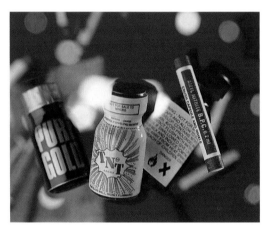

Poppers work by liberation of nitrous oxide which gives short lived euphoria with intensification of current positive emotions

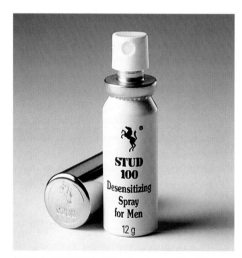

Sprays incorporating lidocaine are used to delay ejaculation

Further reading

Cole M. Sex therapy for individuals. In: Cole M, Dryden W, eds. *Sex therapy in Britain*. Milton Keynes: Open University Press, 1988

Riley AJ, Peet M, Wilson C, eds. *Sexual pharmacology*. Oxford: Oxford Medical Publications, 1993

The pictures of dildos, love balls and breath control games are from the *Regulation* catalogue. The picture of body jewellery is reproduced with permission from Sally Griffin.

Index

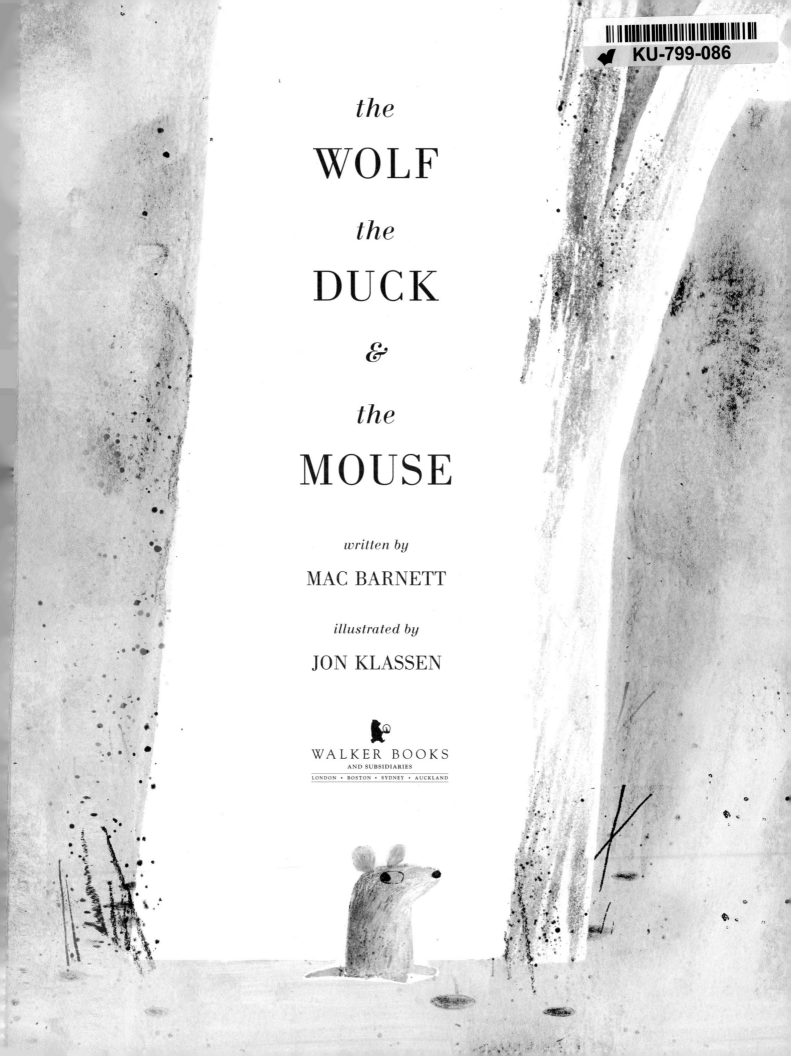

the
WOLF

the
DUCK

&

the
MOUSE

written by

MAC BARNETT

illustrated by

JON KLASSEN

WALKER BOOKS
AND SUBSIDIARIES
LONDON · BOSTON · SYDNEY · AUCKLAND

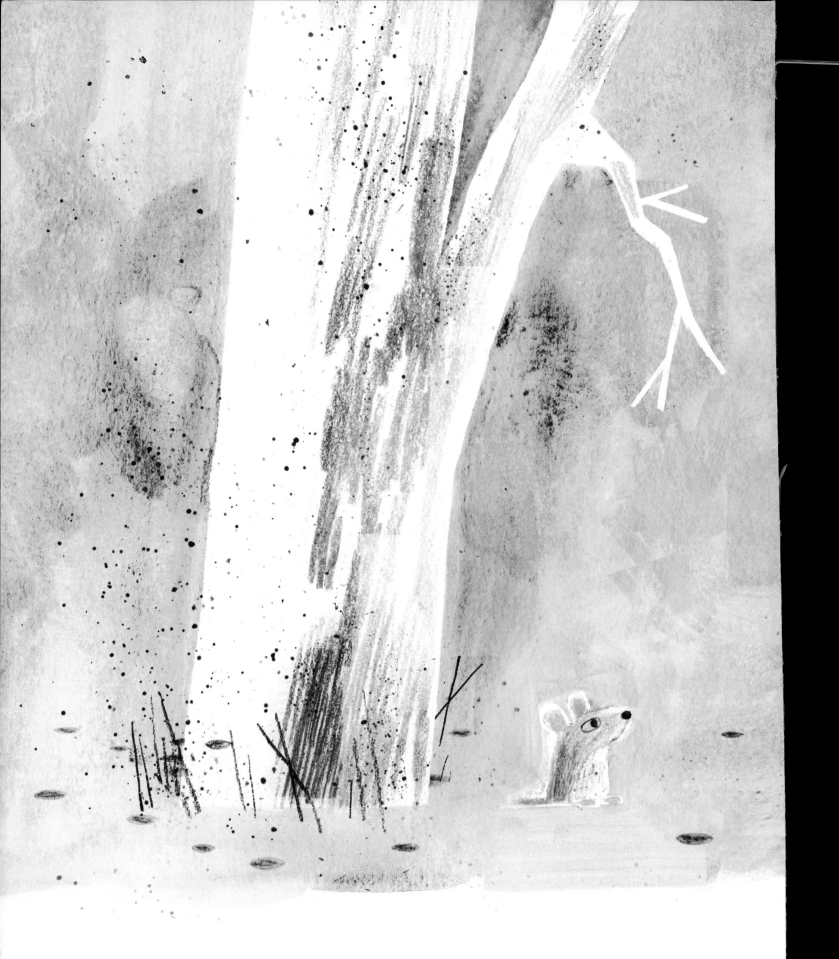

Early one morning, a mouse

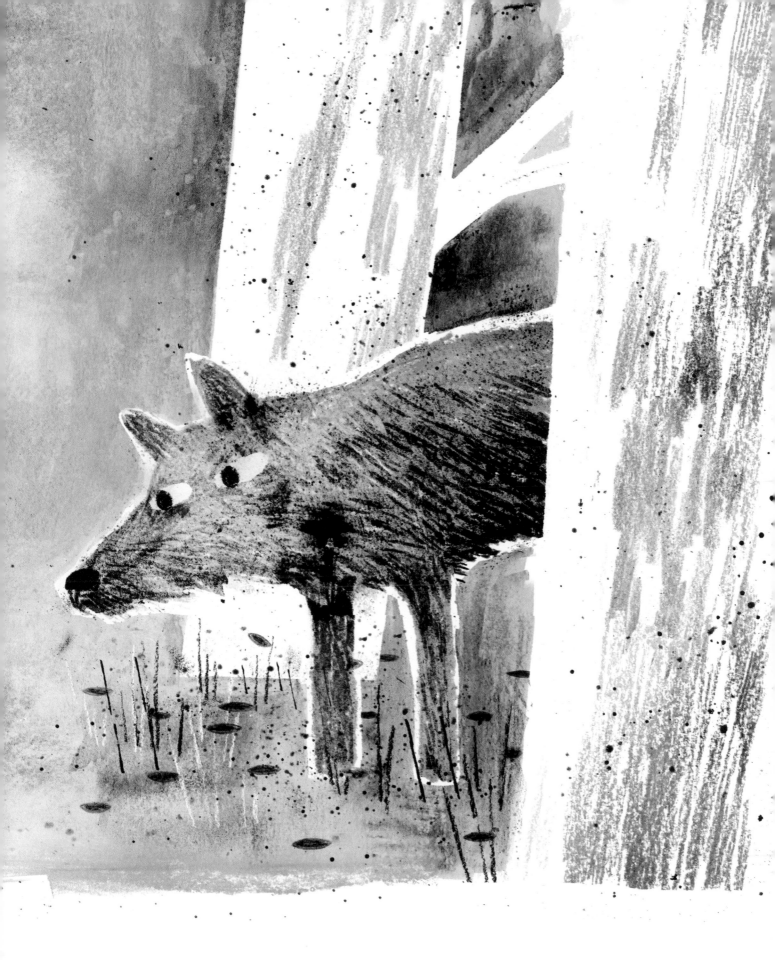

met a wolf,

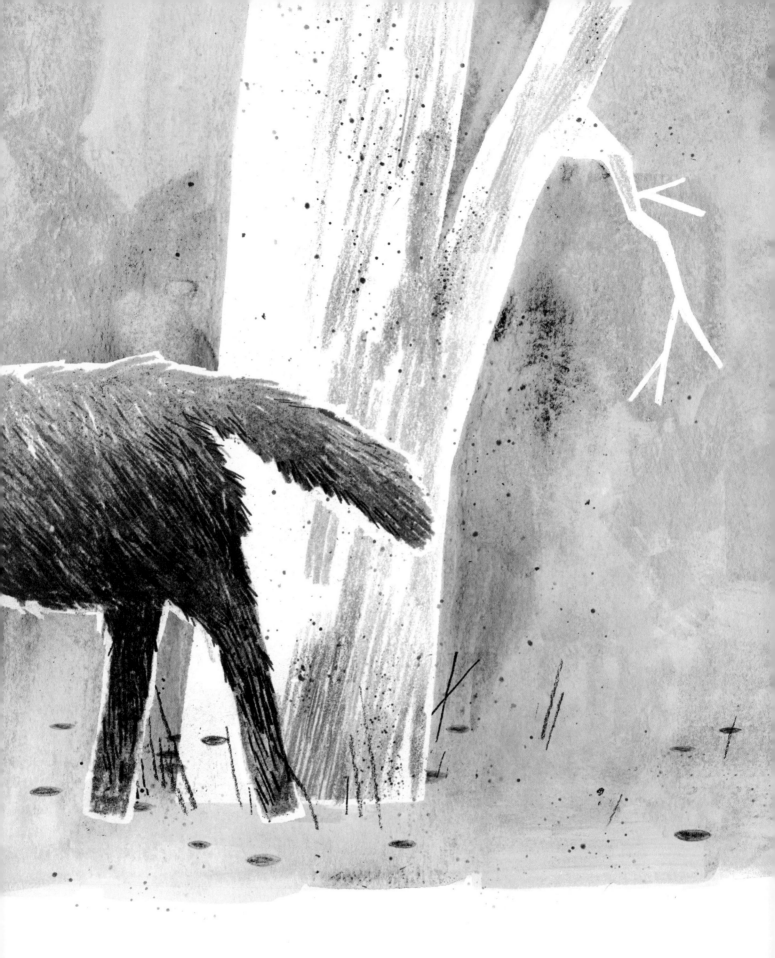

and he was quickly gobbled up.

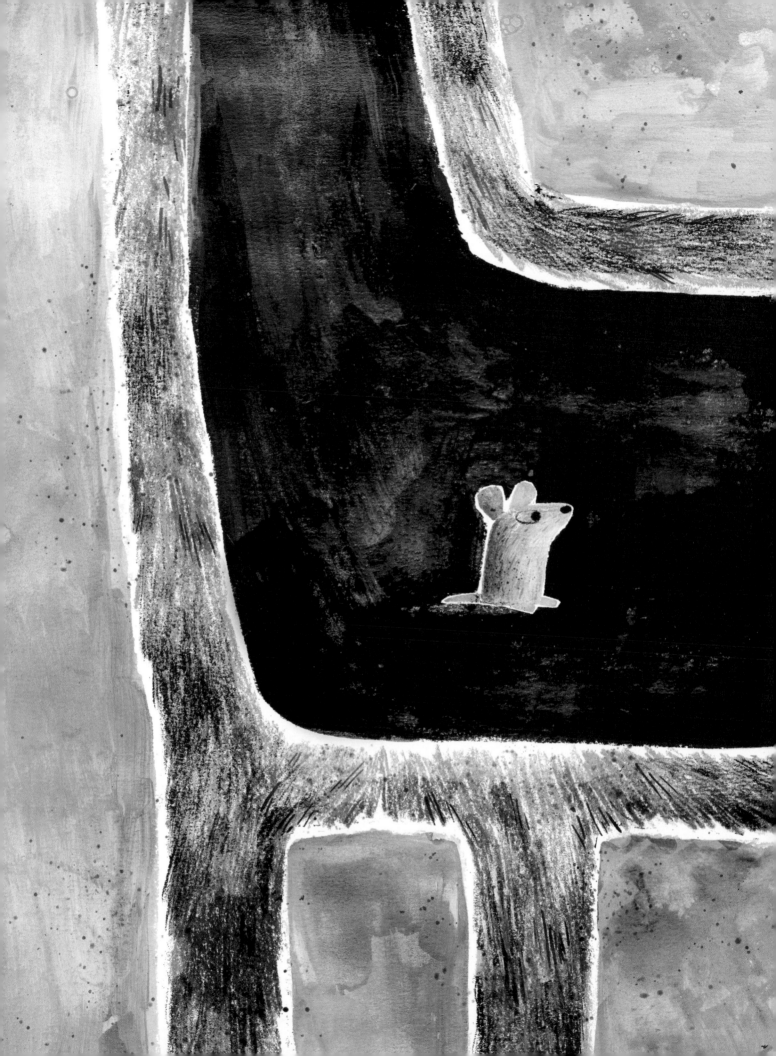

"Oh woe!" said the mouse.

"Oh me! Here I am, caught

in the belly of the beast.

I fear this is the end."

"Be quiet!" someone shouted.

"I'm trying to sleep."

The mouse shrieked, "Who's there?"

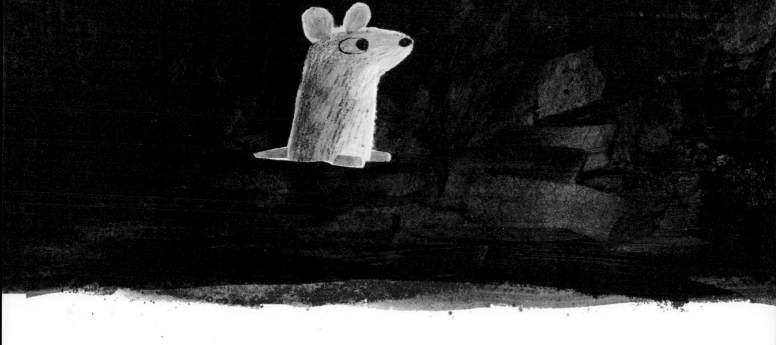

A light was lit. A duck lay in bed.

"Well?" said the duck.

"Oh," said the mouse.

"Is that all?" asked the duck.

"It's the middle of the night."

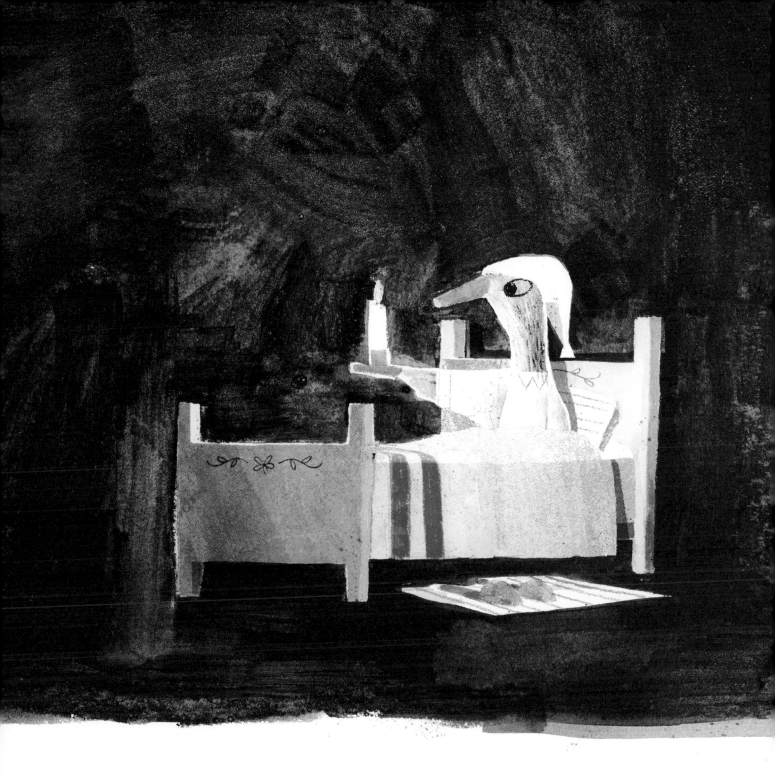

The mouse looked around.

"Well, out there it's morning."

"It is?" said the duck. "It's so hard to tell.

I do wish this belly had a window or two.

In any case, breakfast!"

The meal was delicious.

"Where did you get jam?" the mouse asked.

"And a tablecloth?"

The duck munched a crust.

"You'd be surprised what you find inside
of a wolf."

"It's nice," said the mouse.

"It's home," said the duck.

"You live here?"

"I live well! I may have been swallowed,
but I have no intention of being eaten."

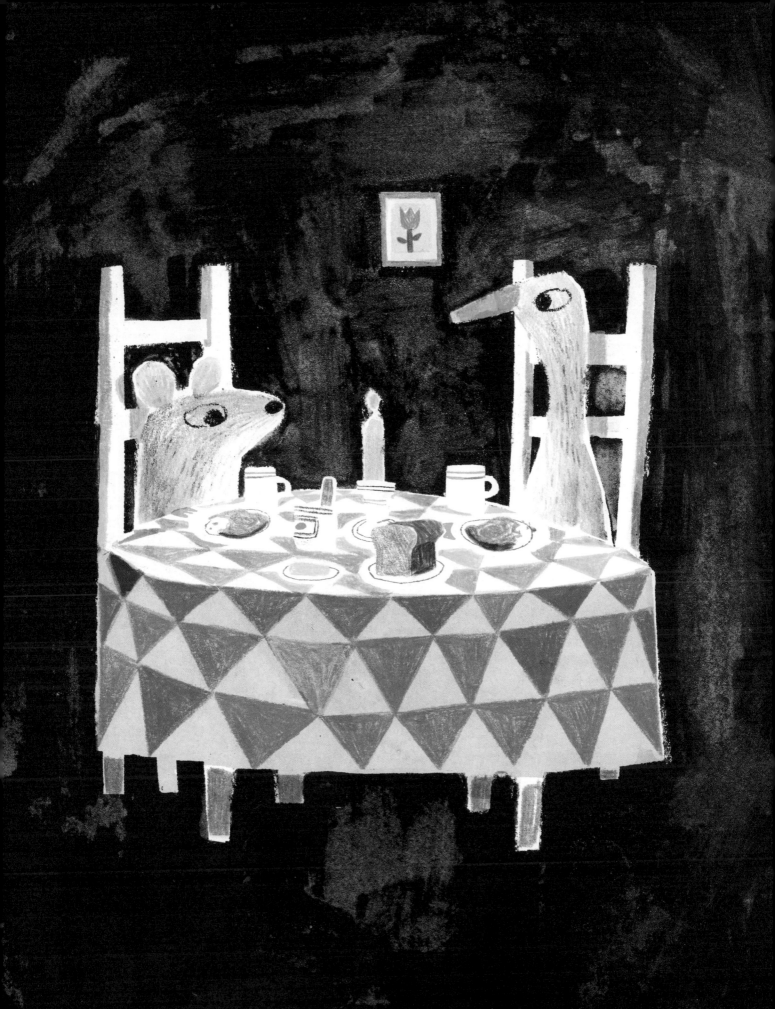

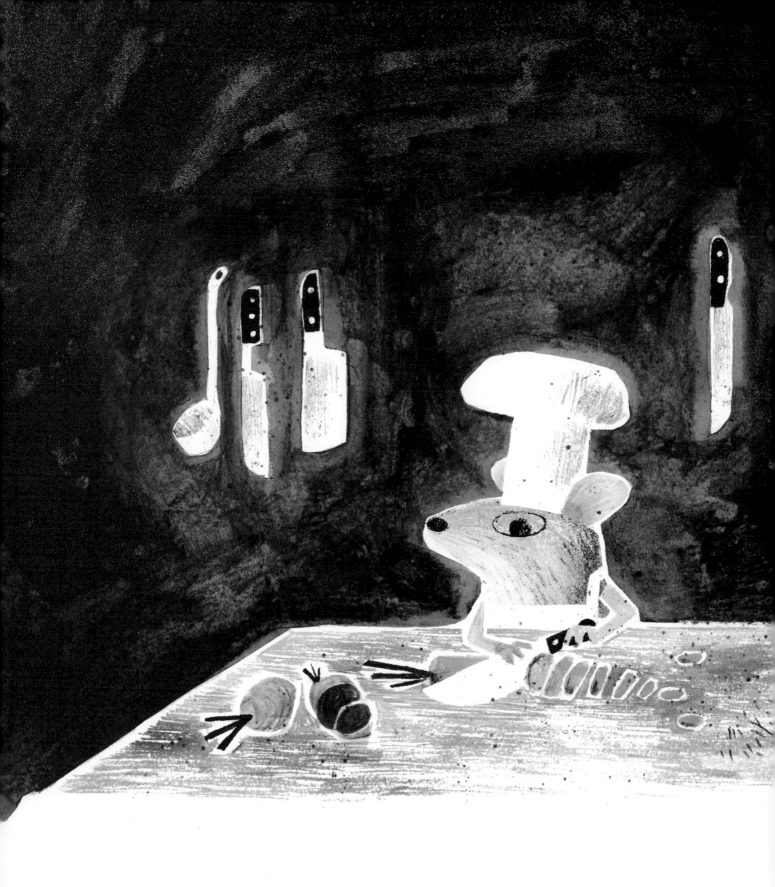

For lunch they made soup.

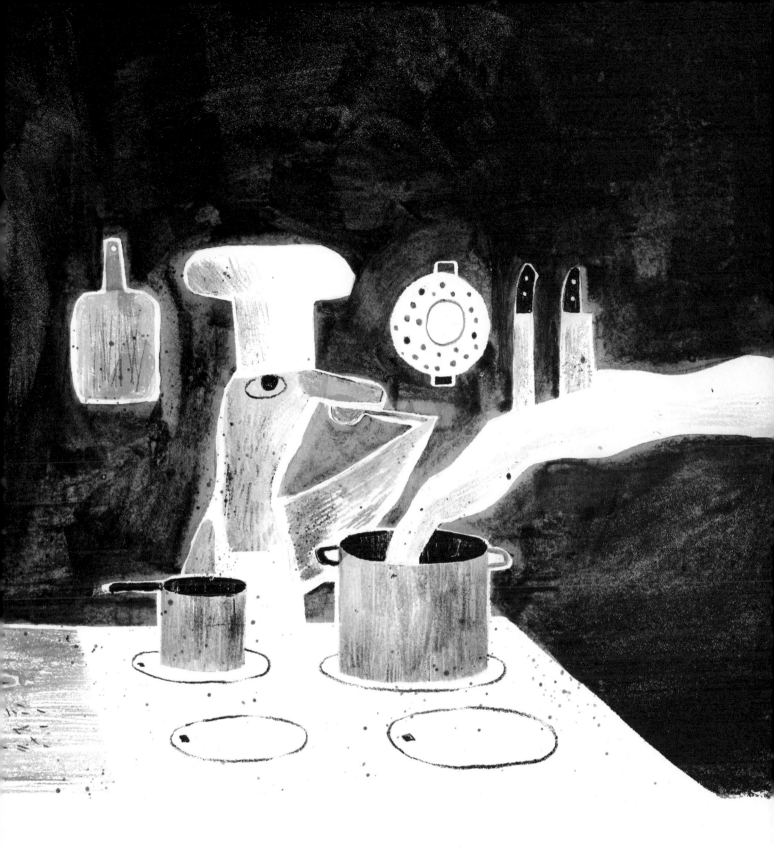

The mouse cleared his throat.

"Do you miss the outside?"

"I do not!" said the duck.

"When I was outside, I was afraid every day
wolves would swallow me up.

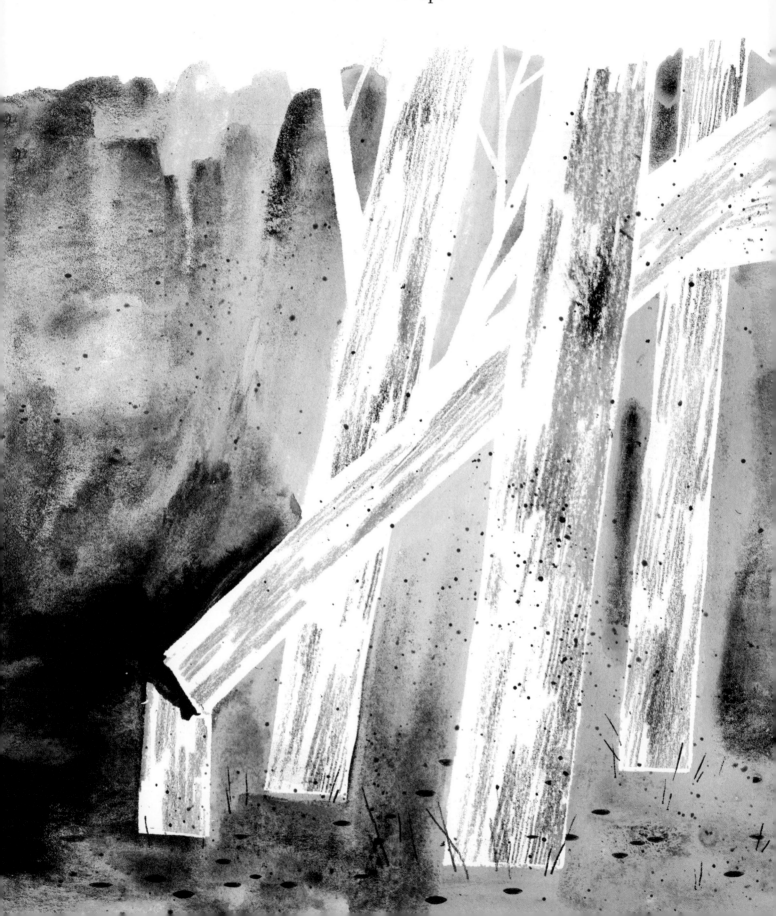

In here, that's no worry."

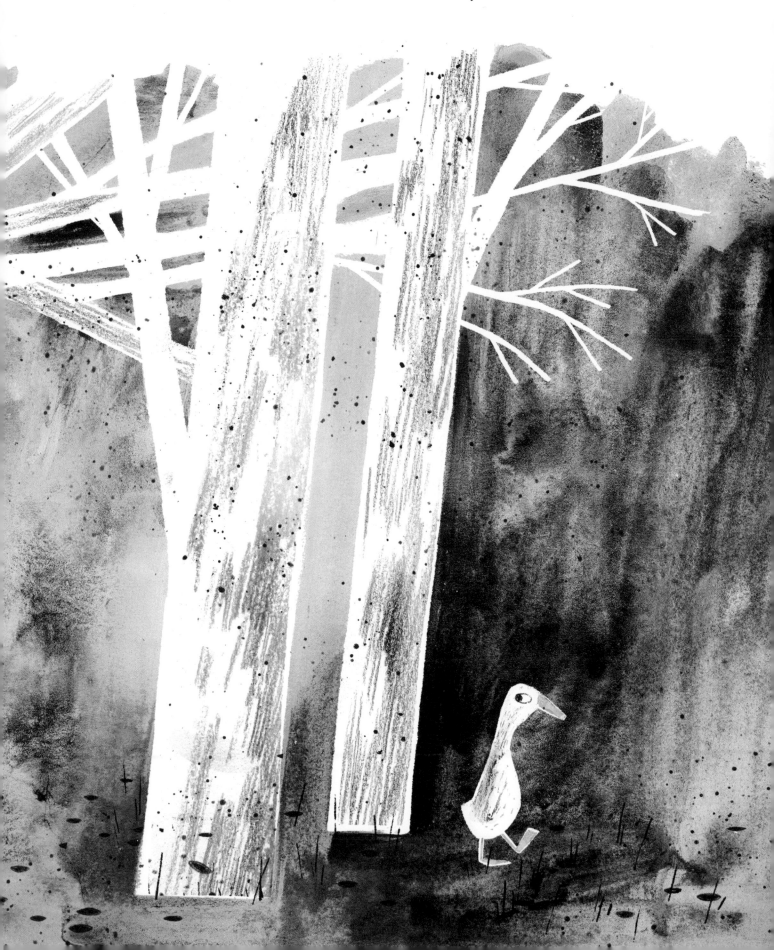

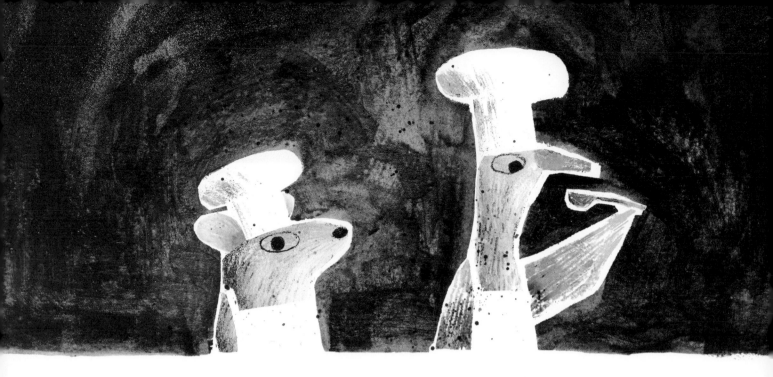

The duck had a point.

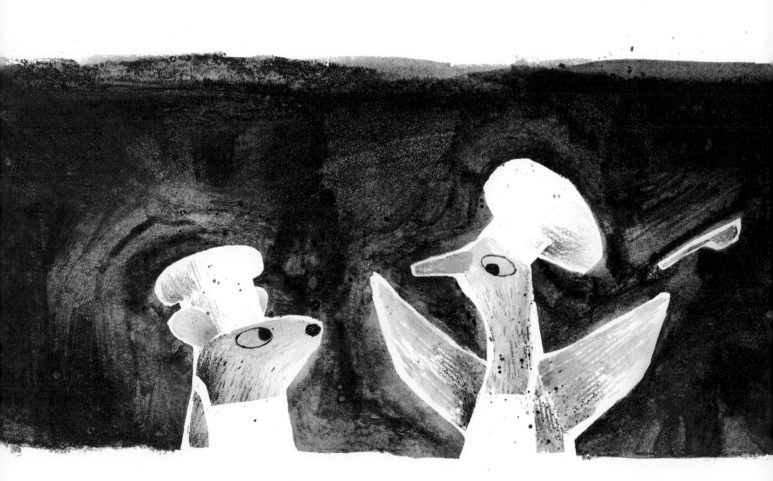

"Can I stay?" the mouse asked.

"Of course!" the duck said.

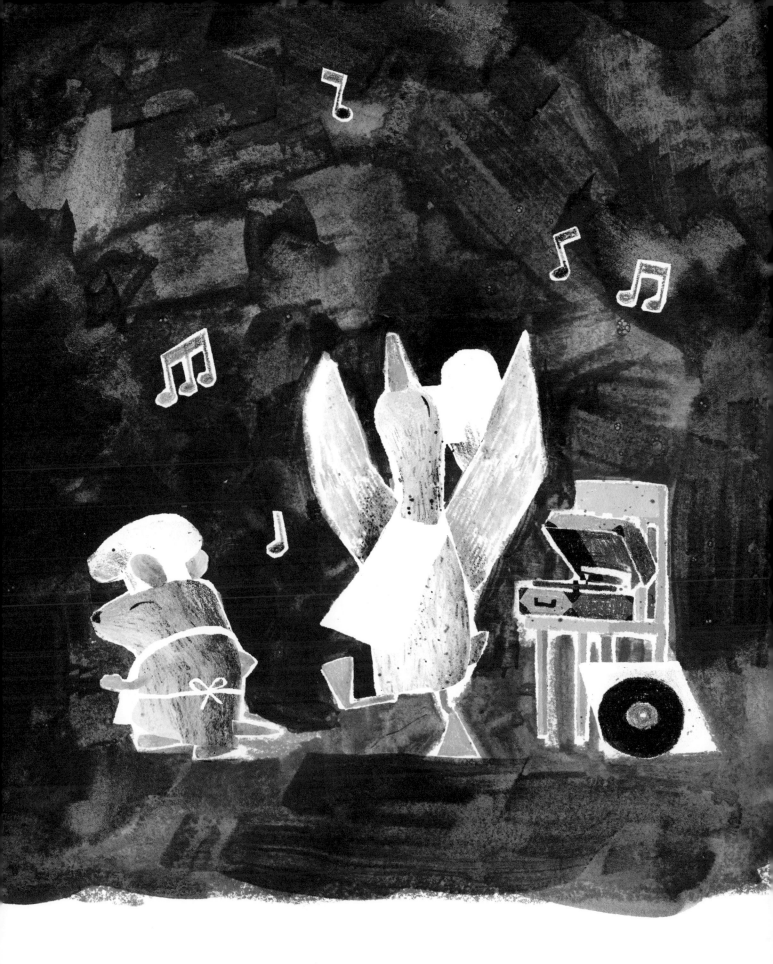

This called for a dance.

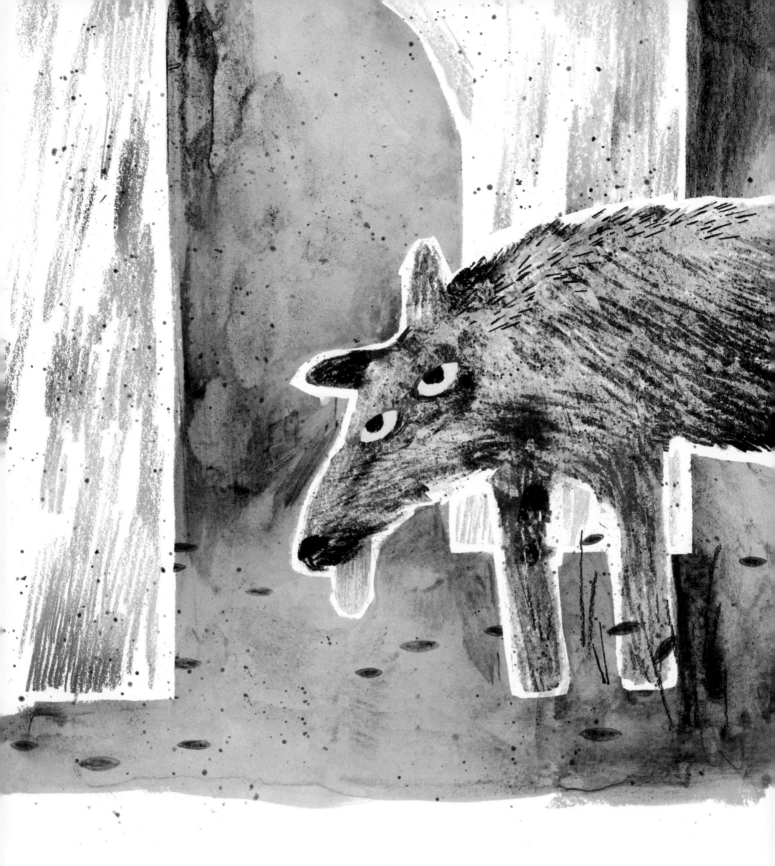

The ruckus inside made the wolf's stomach ache.
"Oh woe!" said the wolf. "Oh shame! Never
have I felt such aching and pain. Surely it must
have been something I ate."

The duck shouted up, "I have a cure!"

"You do?" asked the wolf.

"Yes! An old remedy sure to settle your
tummy. Eat a hunk of good cheese.
And a flagon of wine! And some
beeswax candles."

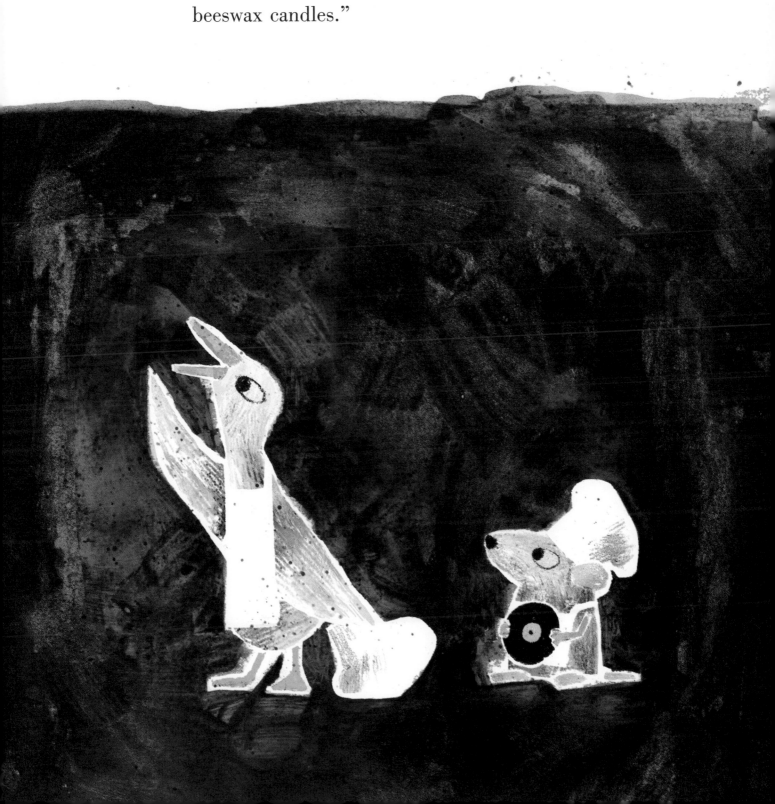

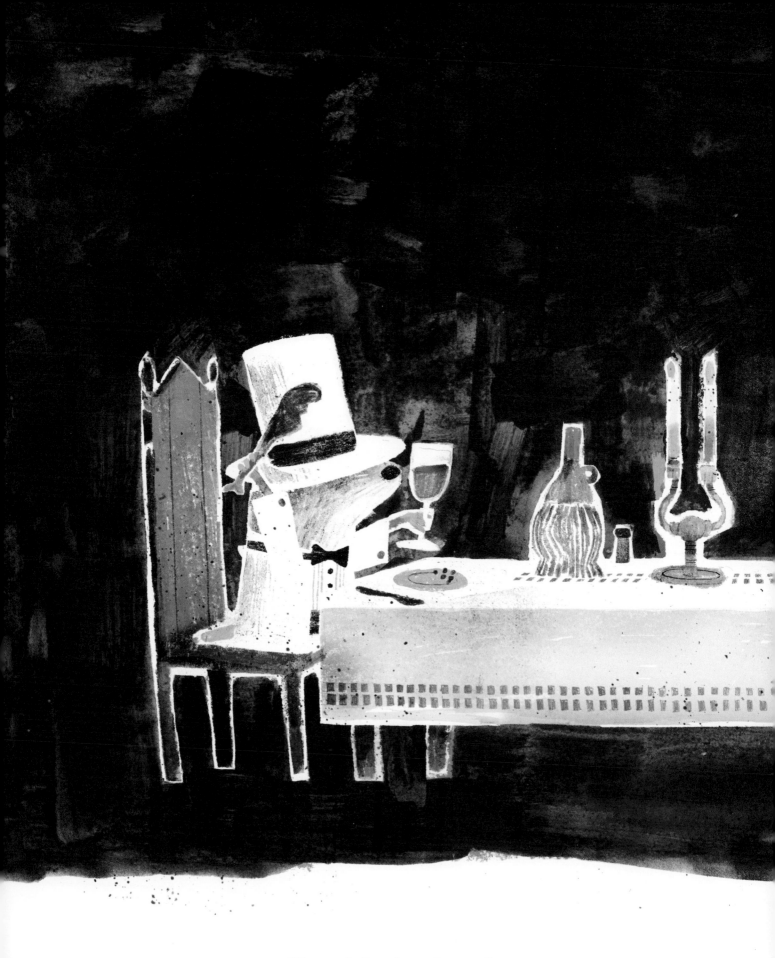

That night they feasted.

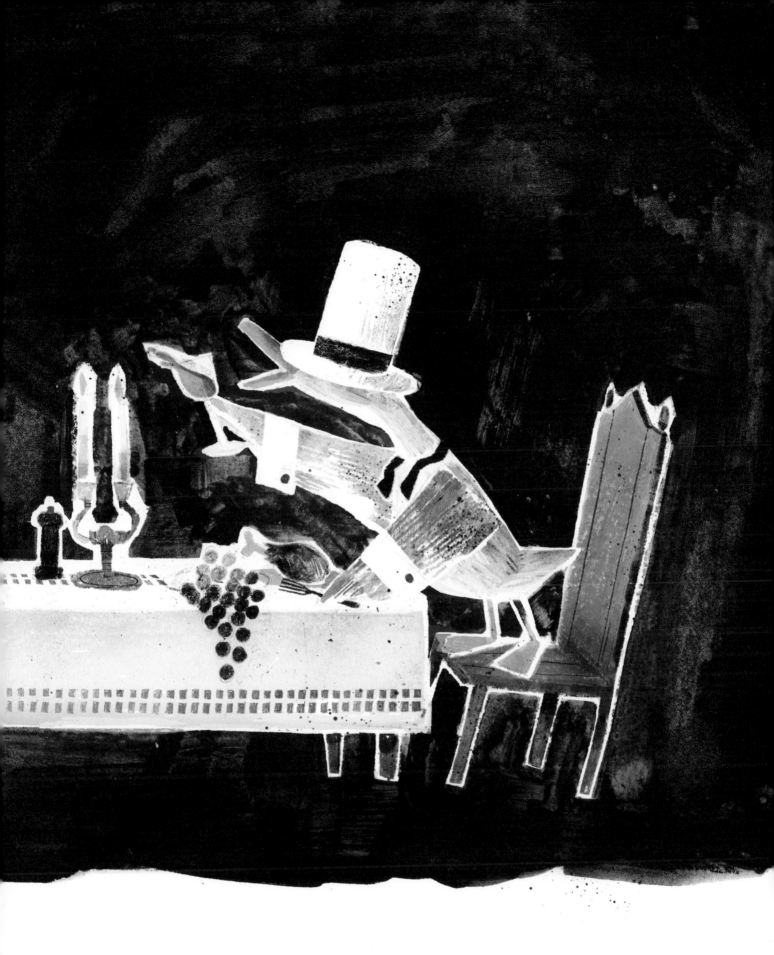

The duck made a toast. "To the health of the wolf!"

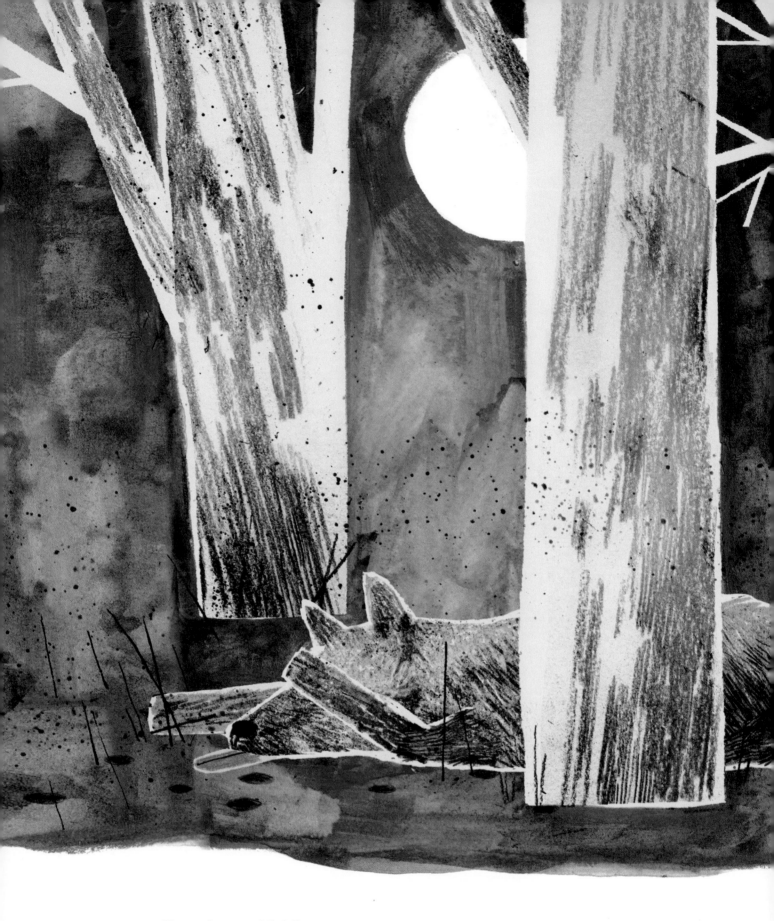

But the wolf felt worse.

"I feel like I'll burst. It hurts just to move."

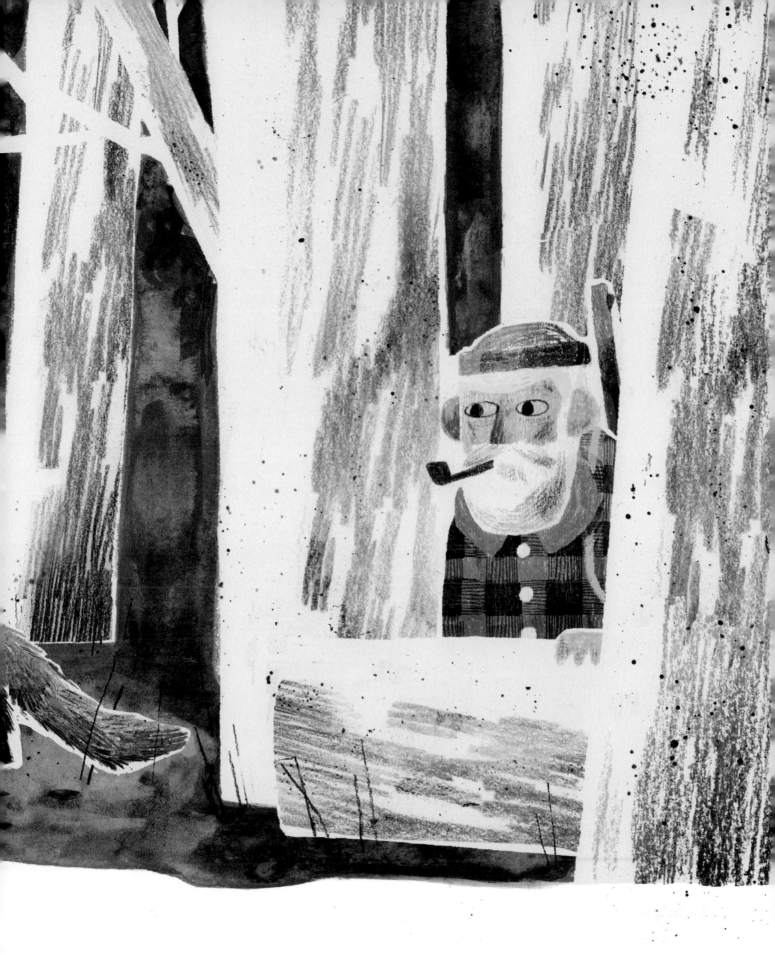

A hunter heard the wolf moan.

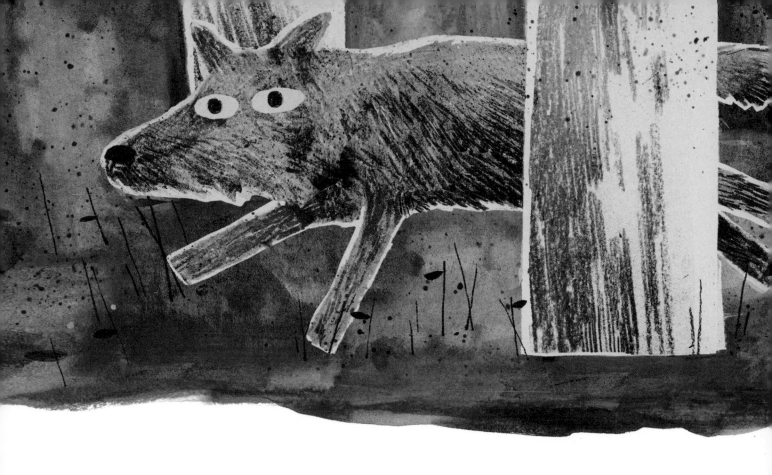

He fired a shot but missed in the dark.

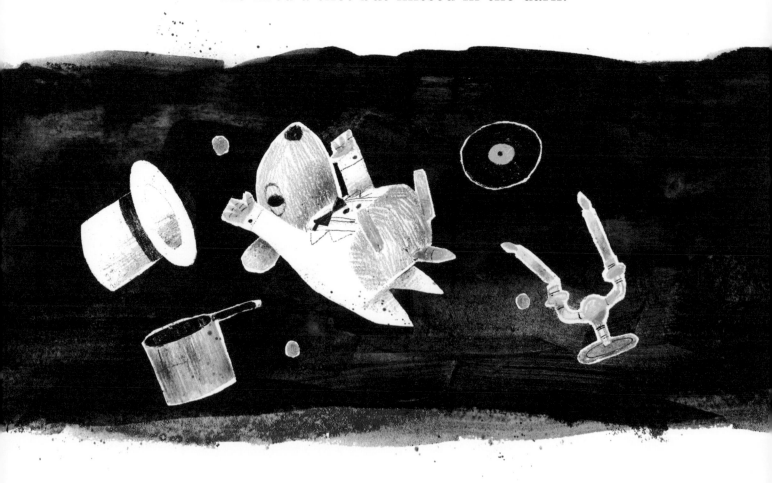

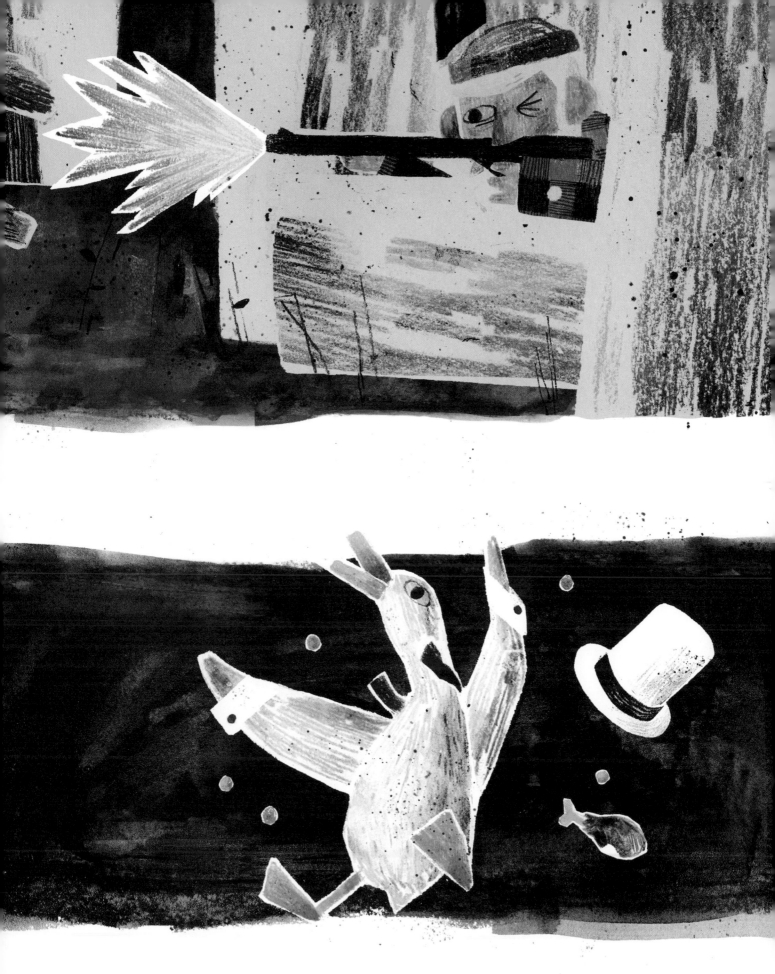

The duck called up, "Run! Run for our lives!"

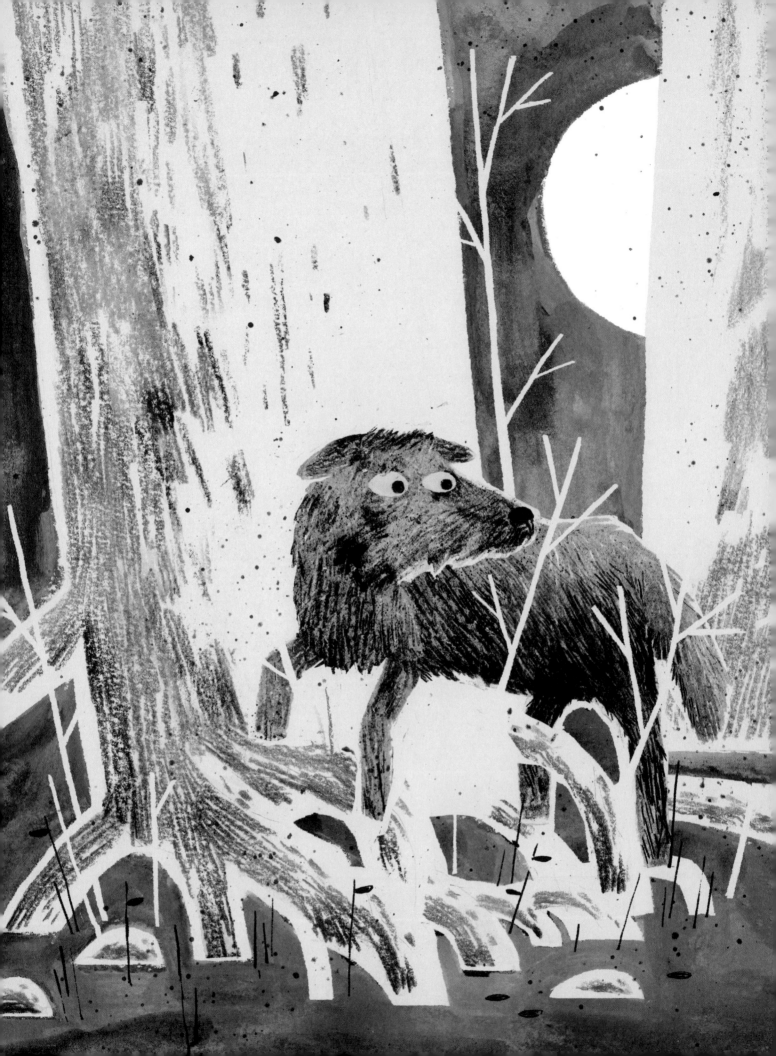

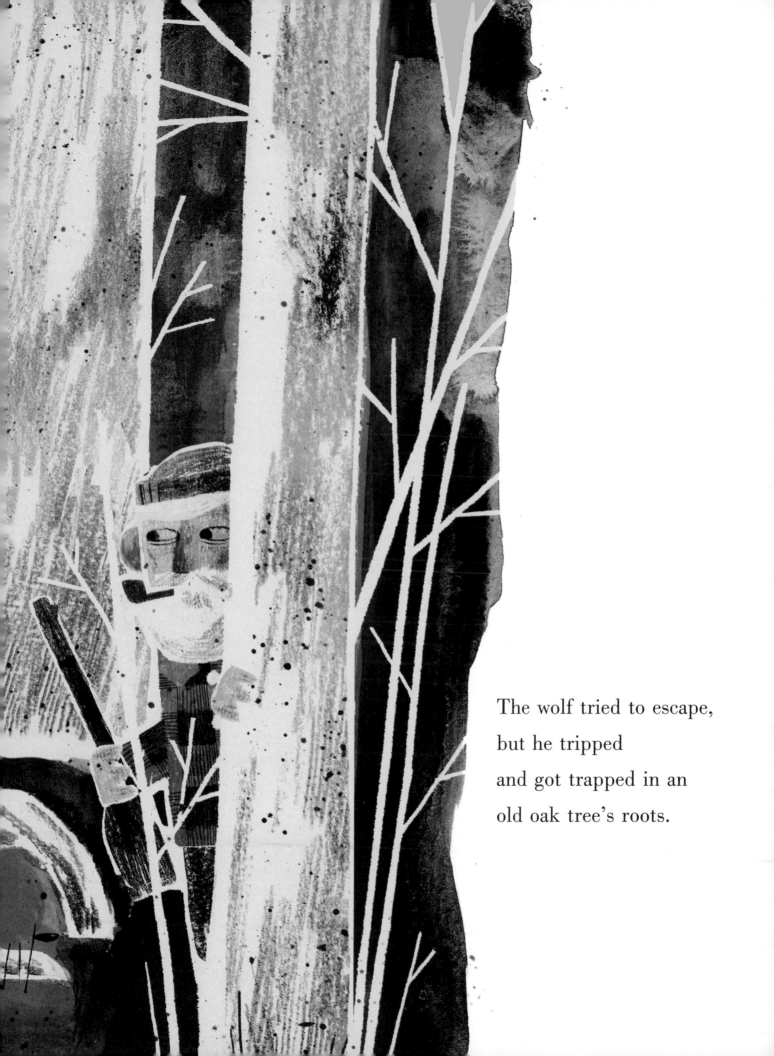

The wolf tried to escape,
but he tripped
and got trapped in an
old oak tree's roots.

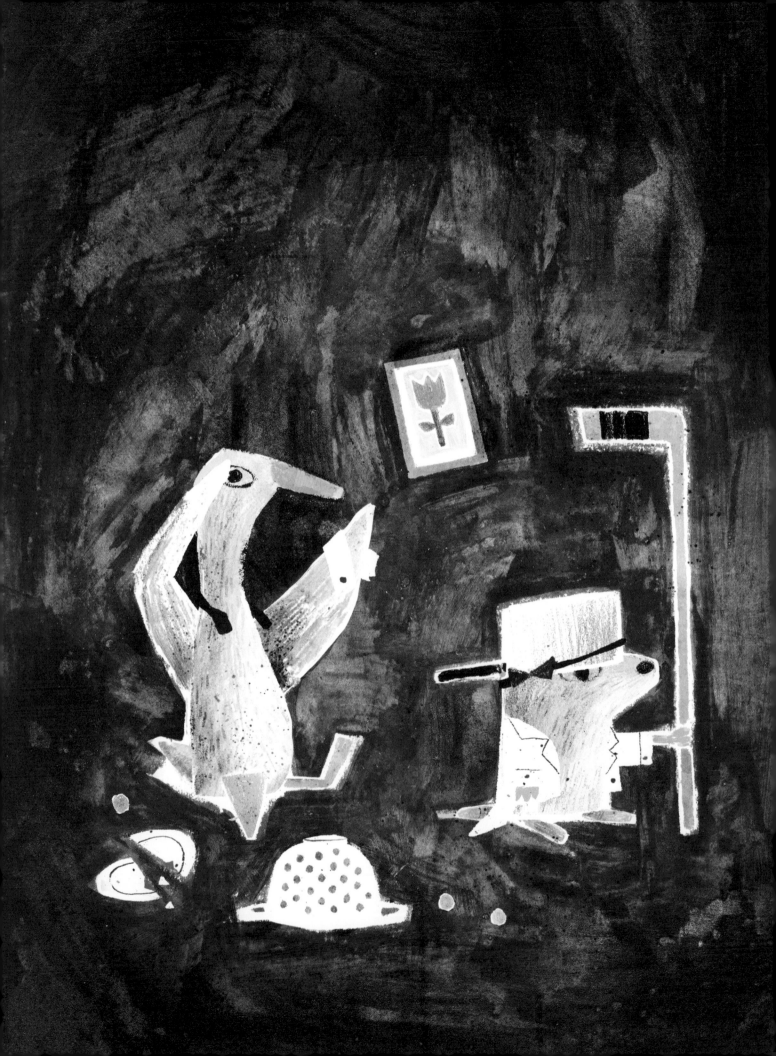

"Oh woe!" said the duck. "Oh doom!
  What can we do? I fear this is the end."
  The mouse stood up.
"We must fight. We must try.
  Tonight we ride to defend our home."

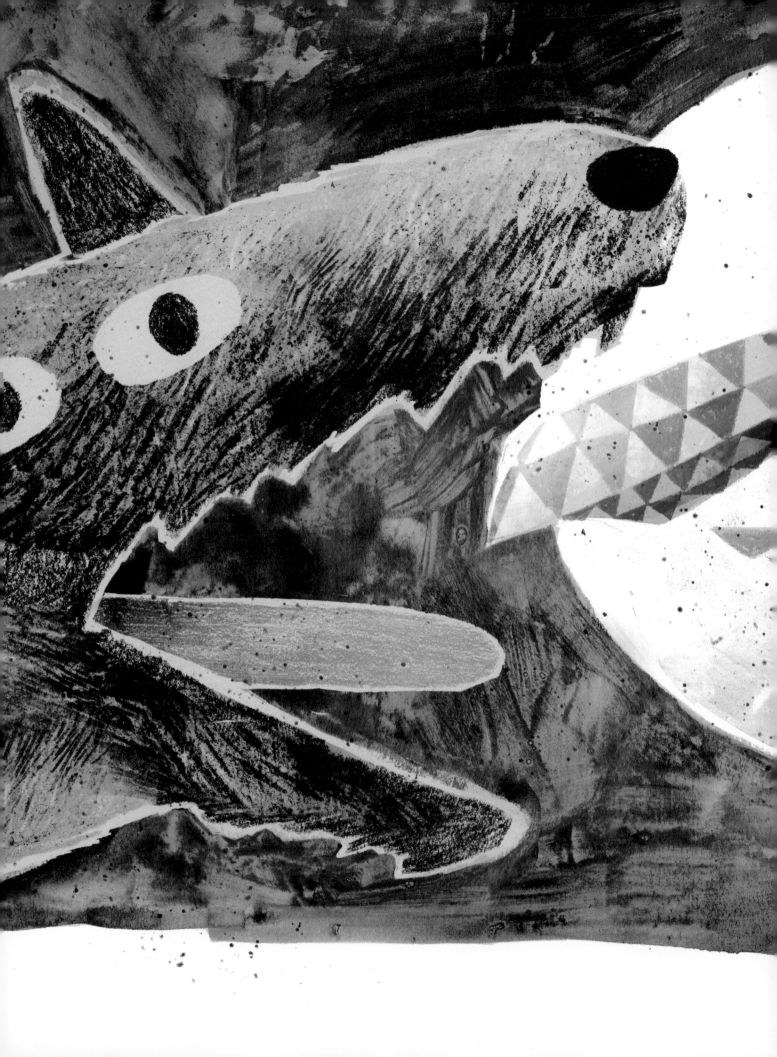

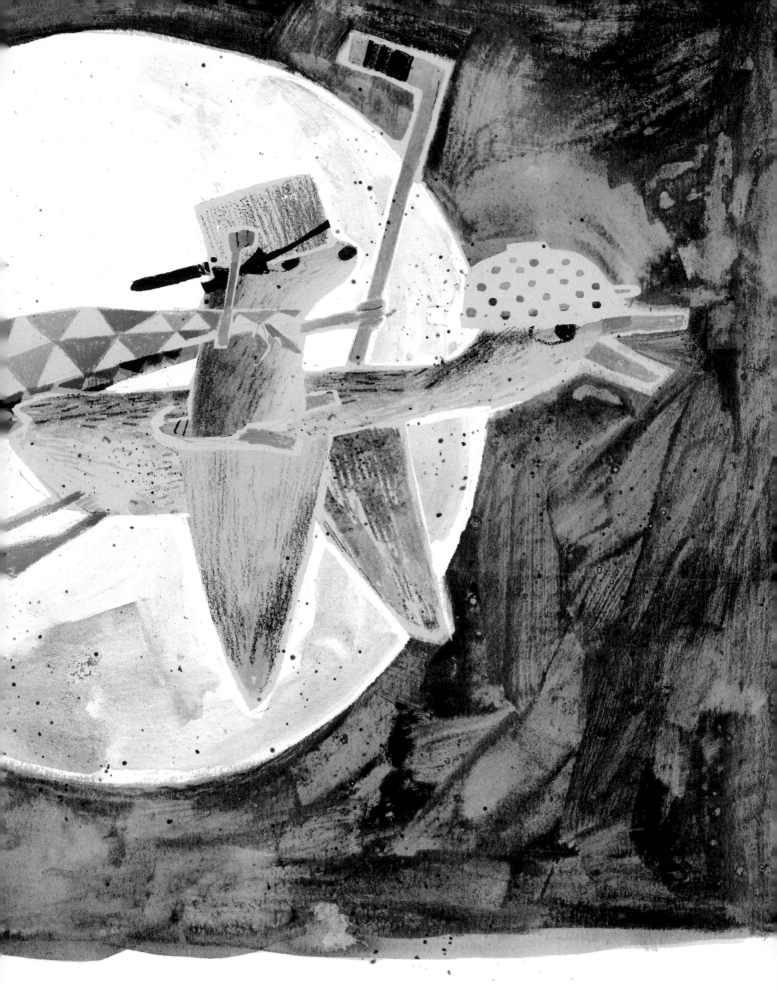

"CHARGE!"

"Oh woe!" said the hunter. "Oh death!
These woods are full of evil and wraiths!"
He fled from the forest and never returned.

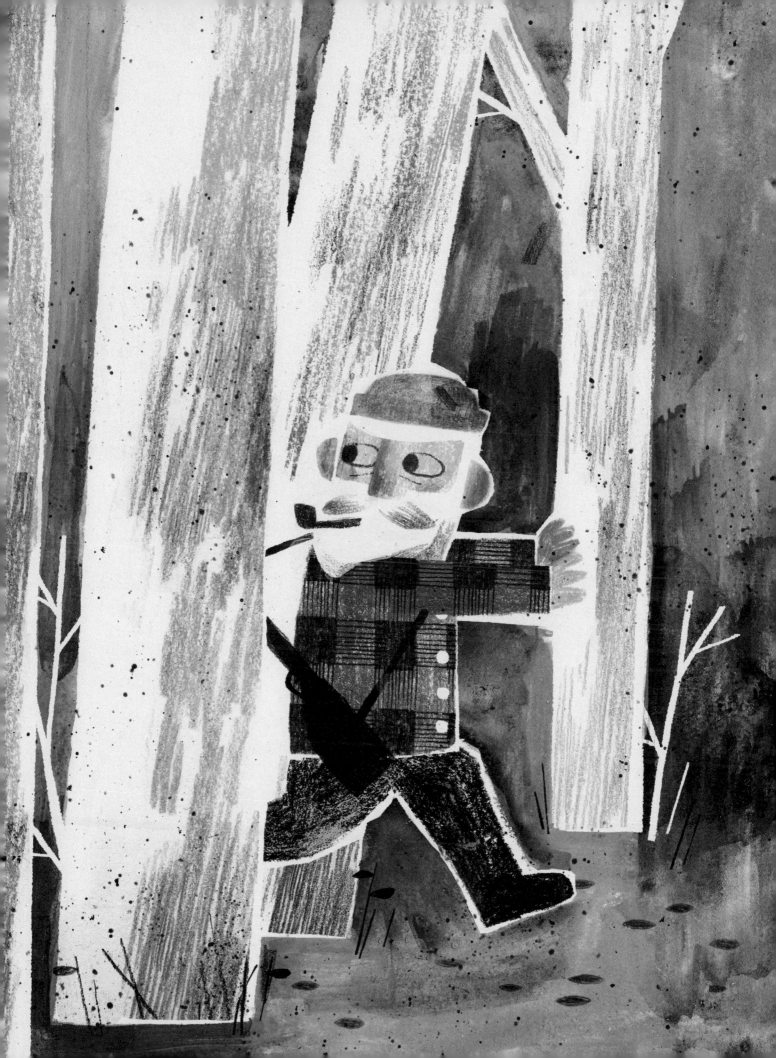

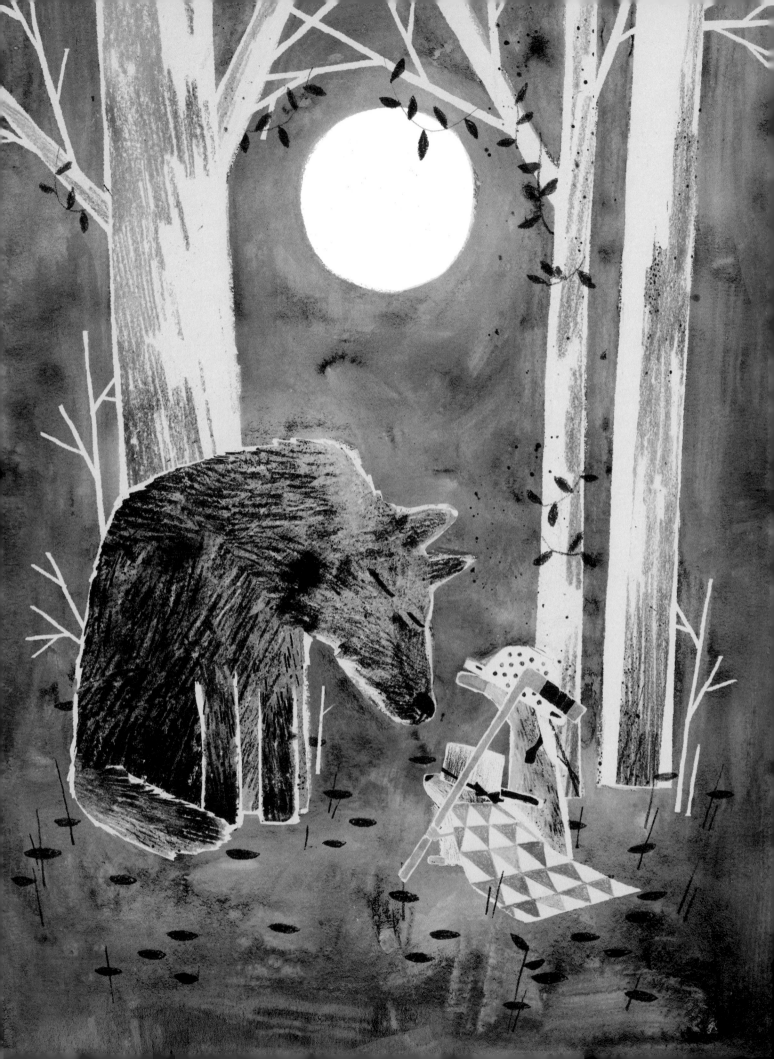

The wolf bowed down
to the duck and the mouse.
"You saved my life
when I thought not
to spare yours.
Ask a favour of me.
I will be glad to grant it."

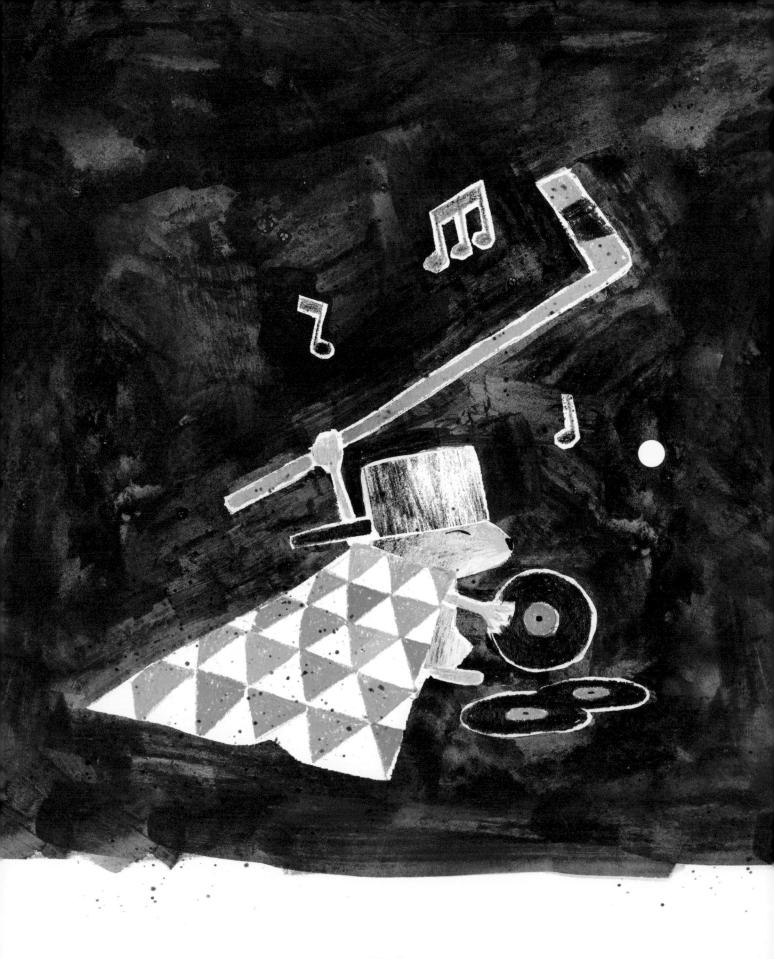

Well,

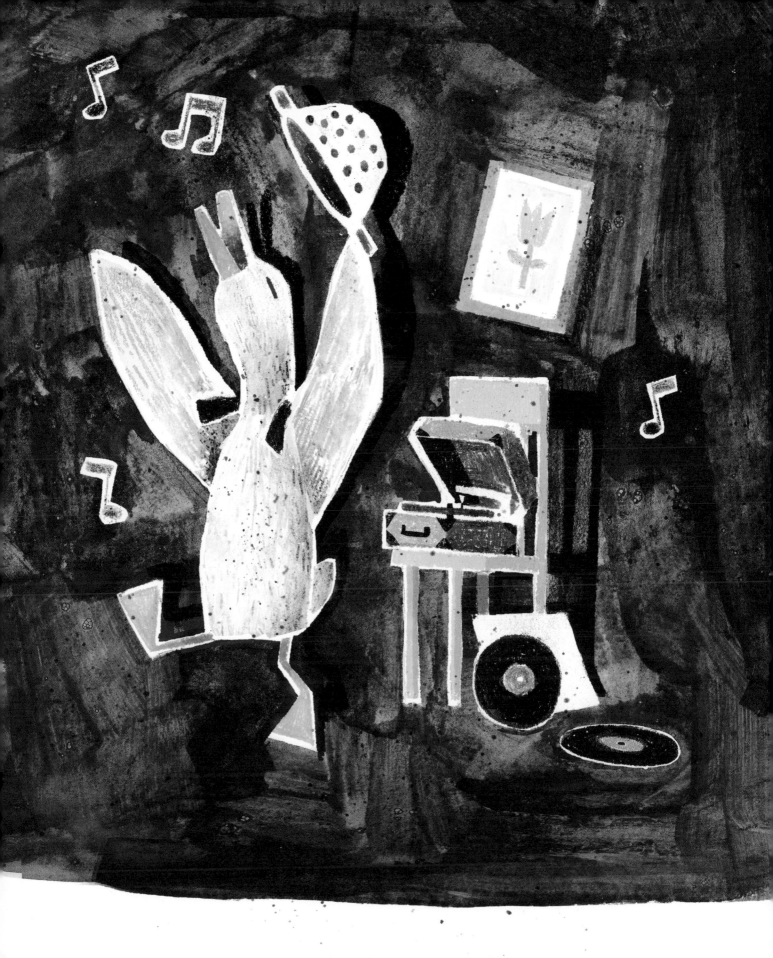

you can guess what they asked for.

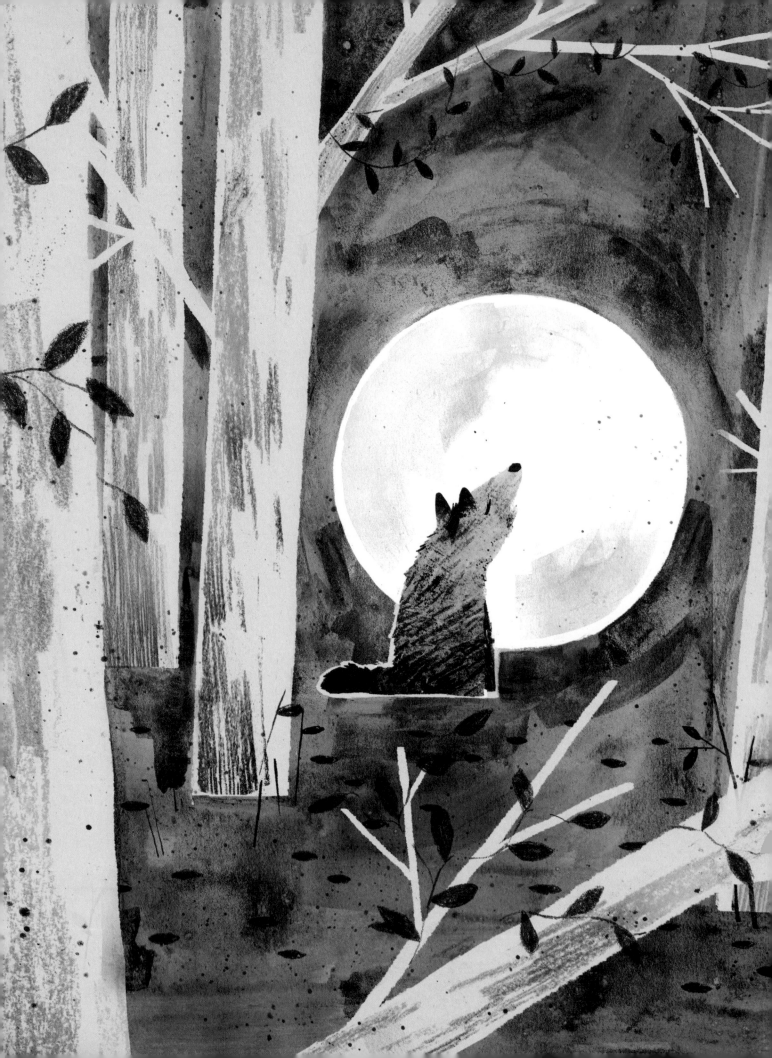